PLANT-BASE POWER BOWLS

COOKBOOK

VEGAN & VEGGIE POWER BOWLS: GLUTEN-FREE, SUGAR-FREE, FODMAP-FRIENDLY & EASY ON YOUR WALLET

DR JANE T. RYAN

Copyright © 2024 by DR Jane T. Ryan

INTRODUCTION

In the bustling landscape of modern culinary delights, where health-conscious choices intertwine with gastronomic innovation, the saga of Plant-Based Power Bowls unfolds. A narrative woven through time, echoing the ancient wisdom of plant-centric nourishment, resurfaces in an era where vitality and sustainability converge.

Picture an ancient garden, where civilizations cultivated the bounty of the earth, recognizing the profound connection between vibrant health and the abundance of plants. Fast-forward to the present day, and witness the resurgence of this timeless ethos in the form of Plant-Based Power Bowls. A culinary evolution rooted in the realization that the harmonious marriage of nutrient-rich ingredients can be both a feast for the senses and a celebration of well-being.

As the world turns toward a greener horizon, these bowls stand as culinary ambassadors, inviting us to indulge in the artistry of assembling flavors, textures, and colors from nature's palette. Each bowl tells a story – a tale of quinoa's ancient whisper, kale's verdant resilience, and the robust character of chickpeas. It's a story that resonates with the modern appetite for conscious living, where the past and present converge on the plate.

In this gastronomic odyssey, Plant-Based Power Bowls transcend mere sustenance; they embody a movement towards vitality and ecological awareness. The ingredients are not just components; they are the protagonists in a narrative that champions health, sustainability, and the exquisite pleasure of savoring the goodness of the earth. Step into this contemporary epic, where history and innovation unite in a delicious symphony – the Plant-Based Power Bowl, a culinary masterpiece for the ages.

WHAT ARE PLANT-BASED POWER BOWLS?

Plant-based power bowls are nutrient-packed meals that showcase a variety of wholesome, plant-derived ingredients in a visually appealing bowl. These bowls typically consist of a combination of grains, vegetables, proteins, and flavorful dressings, offering a balanced and nourishing eating experience.

- Base: The foundation of a plant-based power bowl often includes whole grains like quinoa, brown rice, or farro. These grains include fiber, vital minerals, and complex carbohydrates.
- Vegetables: Colorful and diverse vegetables are a key component, providing a range of vitamins, minerals, and antioxidants. Common choices include leafy greens, bell peppers, tomatoes, carrots, broccoli, and avocado.
- Proteins: Plant-based proteins play a crucial role in these bowls, contributing to satiety and muscle health. Sources may include beans, lentils, chickpeas, tofu, tempeh, or edamame. These ingredients also add texture and flavor diversity.
- Healthy Fats: Avocado, nuts, seeds, or a drizzle of olive oil are often included to provide healthy fats, contributing to the overall nutritional profile and enhancing the meal's taste.
- Dressings and Sauces: Flavorful dressings made from ingredients like tahini, balsamic vinaigrette, or citrus-based sauces add a burst of taste to the bowl. These also serve as a way to tie the various components together.
- Garnishes: Fresh herbs, microgreens, or nutritional yeast can be added as garnishes, not only enhancing the visual appeal but also boosting the nutritional content.
- Customization: One of the strengths of plant-based power bowls is their versatility. Individuals can customize them based on personal preferences, dietary restrictions, or seasonal availability of ingredients.
- Nutrient Density: These bowls are designed to maximize nutrient density, providing a wide array of vitamins, minerals, and phytonutrients. This makes them a great choice for those seeking a well-rounded and health-conscious meal.
- Sustainability: Plant-based power bowls align with sustainability goals, as they often rely on ingredients with a lower environmental impact compared to animal products. Choosing locally sourced and seasonal produce can further enhance the sustainability aspect.
- Meal Prep Friendly: Plant-based power bowls are convenient for meal prep. Preparing components in advance and assembling them when needed allows for quick and easy meals, making them suitable for busy lifestyles.

BENEFITS OF PLANT-BASED EATING

Plant-based eating offers a multitude of health and environmental benefits, making it an increasingly popular choice for many individuals. Here's a detailed exploration of the advantages:

- Nutrient Richness: Plant-based diets are abundant in vitamins, minerals, fiber, and antioxidants derived from fruits, vegetables, whole grains, nuts, and seeds. This nutrient richness contributes to overall health and well-being.

- Heart Health: Plant-based eating is associated with a reduced risk of heart disease. The emphasis on foods like fruits, vegetables, legumes, and nuts helps lower cholesterol levels, blood pressure, and decreases the risk of cardiovascular issues.

- Weight Management: Plant-based diets are often naturally lower in calories and saturated fats, making them conducive to weight management. The high fiber content also promotes a feeling of fullness, reducing the likelihood of overeating.

- Improved Digestive Health: The fiber in plant-based foods promotes healthy digestion by preventing constipation and supporting a diverse and beneficial gut microbiota. This can contribute to a reduced risk of digestive issues and improved overall gut health.

- Cancer Prevention: Plant-based diets may reduce the chance of developing some malignancies, according to several research.

- The abundance of antioxidants and phytochemicals in plant foods may play a role in protecting cells from damage and preventing the development of cancerous cells.

- Blood Sugar Control: Plant-based diets can be effective in managing and preventing type 2 diabetes. The complex carbohydrates found in whole plant foods have a gentler impact on blood sugar levels compared to refined carbohydrates.

- Inflammation Reduction: Numerous illnesses, including as arthritis and several forms of cancer, are associated with chronic inflammation.

- Plant-based diets, rich in anti-inflammatory compounds, can help reduce inflammation and promote overall health.

- Kidney Health: For individuals with kidney issues, a plant-based diet may be beneficial. It can help manage blood pressure and reduce the load on the kidneys by providing a lower intake of certain minerals and compounds.

- Environmental Sustainability: Plant-based eating is recognized for its lower environmental impact compared to diets high in animal products. Producing plant foods generally requires fewer resources like water and land, and it generates fewer greenhouse gas emissions.

- Animal care: Adopting a plant-based diet is consistent with moral principles pertaining to the care of animals By reducing or eliminating animal product consumption, individuals contribute to the ethical treatment of animals in the food industry.

- Longevity: Some studies suggest that plant-based diets are associated with increased longevity. The combination of disease prevention, weight management, and overall health benefits may contribute to a longer and healthier life.

1

Essential Components of a Power Bowl

Base: Grains and Greens

- Base: Grains and Greens are foundational components of a nutritious Power Bowl, providing essential elements for a well-rounded and satisfying meal. Grains, such as quinoa, brown rice, or farro, serve as a hearty and fiber-rich base, offering complex carbohydrates that provide sustained energy. These grains also contribute essential minerals like iron and magnesium.

Greens, such as kale, spinach, or arugula, form the nutrient-packed foundation of the bowl, supplying an array of vitamins, including A, C, and K. Dark leafy greens are rich in antioxidants and contribute to overall health. They also bring a refreshing crunch and vibrant color to the bowl.

In combination, grains and greens create a balanced source of carbohydrates, fiber, and micronutrients. The fiber content aids in digestion and promotes a feeling of fullness, while the carbohydrates fuel the body with energy. Additionally, the micronutrients from greens play a crucial role in supporting immune function, bone health, and skin integrity.

To enhance the nutritional profile of the bowl, one can further customize by incorporating various grains like quinoa for complete protein or whole wheat for added fiber. Mixing different greens adds diversity in nutrients, ensuring a broad spectrum of vitamins and minerals.

- The Base: Grains and Greens in a Power Bowl not only contributes to the nutritional density of the meal but also provides a versatile canvas for the addition of protein, healthy fats, and flavorful toppings. This dynamic combination allows for endless variations, making Power Bowls a delicious and health-conscious choice for a well-rounded meal.

Protein Sources

Protein sources are a pivotal component of a Power Bowl, contributing to muscle maintenance, satiety, and overall nutritional balance. Incorporating diverse and high-quality proteins enhances the bowl's nutrient profile, making it a satisfying and wholesome meal.

- Lean Animal Proteins: Chicken breast, turkey, and lean cuts of beef are excellent sources of complete protein, supplying essential amino acids crucial for muscle repair and overall body function.

Fish, such as salmon or tuna, not only provides protein but also delivers omega-3 fatty acids, promoting heart health and reducing inflammation.

- Plant-Based Proteins: Legumes like chickpeas, black beans, and lentils offer a plant-based protein source rich in fiber, iron, and various vitamins. They supply steady energy and aid in the sensation of fullness. Tofu and tempeh are versatile soy-based proteins that absorb flavors well, adding a meaty texture to the bowl. They are particularly beneficial for those following a vegetarian or vegan diet.
- Quinoa and Whole Grains Quinoa stands out as a complete protein, containing all essential amino acids. It serves as both a base and a protein source, making it an ideal choice for a Power Bowl.

Brown rice, farro, and other whole grains contribute not only protein but also complex carbohydrates, offering a steady release of energy.

- Dairy and Dairy Alternatives: Greek yogurt and cottage cheese provide a creamy texture and a significant protein boost. They also deliver calcium for bone health.

Plant-based alternatives like almond or soy yogurt offer protein options for those with dietary preferences or restrictions.

Including a variety of protein sources ensures a comprehensive intake of amino acids and other essential nutrients. The combination of grains, greens, and proteins in a Power Bowl creates a well-rounded meal that supports overall health, muscle maintenance, and sustained energy levels. Customizing protein sources based on dietary preferences and requirements allows for endless possibilities in creating a delicious and nutritious Power Bowl.

Healthy Fats

Healthy fats play a crucial role in the composition of a Power Bowl, contributing to flavor, satiety, and overall nutritional balance. Including a variety of nutrient-dense fats enhances the meal's palatability and provides essential fatty acids necessary for various bodily functions.

- Avocado: Avocado is a nutrient powerhouse, offering heart-healthy monounsaturated fats. It adds a creamy texture to the bowl while providing fiber, potassium, and vitamins such as B6, C, and E.
- Nuts and Seeds: Almonds, walnuts, chia seeds, and flaxseeds are excellent sources of healthy fats, omega-3 fatty acids, and antioxidants. They add a satisfying crunch to the bowl while contributing essential nutrients.
- Olive Oil: Extra virgin olive oil is a staple for dressing a Power Bowl. It contains monounsaturated fats and polyphenols, providing anti-inflammatory benefits and enhancing the absorption of fat-soluble vitamins.
- Fatty Fish: Salmon, mackerel, and sardines are rich in omega-3 fatty acids, promoting heart health and supporting cognitive function. Grilled or baked fish can be a flavorful and nutritious addition to a Power Bowl.
- Coconut: Coconut, whether in the form of shredded coconut, coconut oil, or coconut milk, contributes a unique flavor and texture. While high in saturated fats, coconut also contains medium-chain triglycerides (MCTs) that may have metabolic benefits.
- Nut Butters: Peanut butter, almond butter, or other nut butters provide a tasty source of healthy fats and protein. They can be drizzled over the bowl or incorporated into dressings for added richness.

Balancing healthy fats in a Power Bowl enhances the absorption of fat-soluble vitamins (A, D, E, K) and helps maintain a feeling of fullness. The combination of grains, greens, proteins, and healthy fats creates a well-rounded and satisfying meal that supports overall health and provides sustained energy. Customizing the types and amounts of healthy fats allows for flexibility in creating diverse and flavorful Power Bowl variations.

Flavorful Dressings and Sauces

Flavorful dressings and sauces are the crowning touch in elevating the taste and enjoyment of a Power Bowl. Not only do they add zest and complexity, but they also contribute to the overall harmony of the meal, tying together the diverse components. Here are some essential elements of flavorful dressings and sauces:

- Vinaigrettes: A classic vinaigrette combines olive oil, vinegar (such as balsamic or red wine vinegar), Dijon mustard, and seasonings. This tangy concoction not only enhances the flavors but also provides healthy fats from olive oil.
- Tahini-Based Dressings: Tahini, made from ground sesame seeds, forms a rich and creamy base for dressings. Combining tahini with lemon juice, garlic, and a touch of honey or maple syrup creates a versatile sauce that complements both grains and greens.
- Citrus-Based Sauces:
- Fresh citrus juices, like lemon, lime, or orange, can be used to create light and refreshing dressings. Citrus adds brightness to the bowl, and the acidity helps balance the richness of other components.
- Yogurt-Based Sauces: Greek yogurt or plant-based yogurt alternatives serve as a base for creamy and tangy dressings. Mixing them with herbs, garlic, and lemon juice creates a delightful sauce that pairs well with various ingredients.
- Soy-Based Dressings: Soy sauce or tamari, combined with sesame oil, garlic, and ginger, creates a savory and umami-rich dressing. This is particularly suitable for bowls with Asian-inspired flavors.
- Herb-infused Dressings: Fresh herbs like basil, cilantro, parsley, or mint can be blended with olive oil, garlic, and lemon to create a vibrant and aromatic dressing. Herb-infused options add a burst of freshness to the bowl.

Customizing dressings and sauces allows for endless variations, catering to individual taste preferences. These additions not only enhance the flavor but also provide a means to incorporate additional nutrients and antioxidants. Choosing homemade dressings with high-quality ingredients ensures control over the flavor profile and the avoidance of unnecessary additives. Ultimately, flavorful dressings and sauces are the creative elements that transform a Power Bowl into a delicious and satisfying culinary experience.

2

Breakfast Bowls

Energizing Quinoa and Berry Bowl

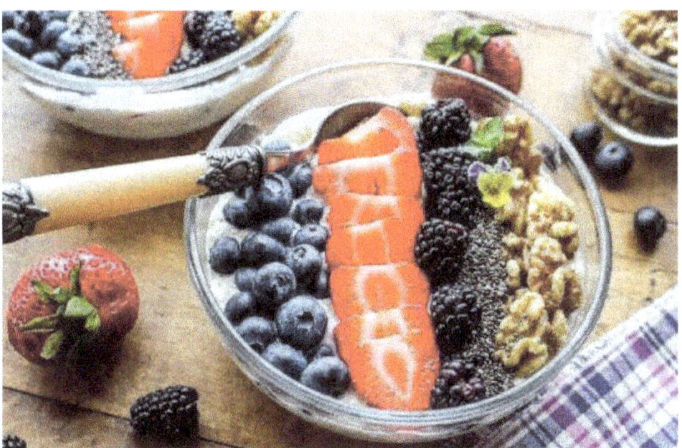

Ingredients:

- 1 cup quinoa
- 2 cups mixed berries (strawberries, blueberries, raspberries)
- 1/4 cup chopped nuts (almonds, walnuts)
- 1 tablespoon chia seeds
- 1 tablespoon honey
- 1 cup Greek yogurt
- 1 teaspoon vanilla extract
- Fresh mint leaves for garnish

Procedure:

- Rinse quinoa thoroughly and cook according to package instructions.
- In a bowl, mix cooked quinoa with Greek yogurt and vanilla extract.
- Top with mixed berries, chopped nuts, chia seeds, and drizzle honey.
- Garnish with fresh mint leaves.

Time of Preparation:

- Approximately 20-25 minutes.

Tips and Tricks:

- Fluff quinoa with a fork after cooking for a light texture.
- Customize with additional toppings like sliced bananas or coconut flakes.
- Adjust honey quantity based on personal sweetness preference.

Nutritional Value per Serving:

- Calories: ~350 kcal
- Protein: ~15g
- Fiber: ~8g
- Healthy Fats: ~10g

Health Benefits:

- Quinoa provides complete protein and essential amino acids.
- Berries are rich in antioxidants and vitamins.
- Nuts add healthy fats and crunch, aiding satiety.

Packaging and Storing:

- Store in airtight containers in the refrigerator for up to 2 days.
- Keep berries separate if preparing in advance to maintain freshness.

Precautions:

- Check for nut allergies before adding nuts.
- Ensure proper rinsing of quinoa to remove bitterness.
- Adjust portion sizes based on individual dietary needs.

Post-Caution:

- Consume within 2 days to retain freshness.

- Refrigerate promptly to avoid bacterial growth.

- Be mindful of portion control for a balanced diet.

Avocado and Sweet Potato Breakfast Bowl

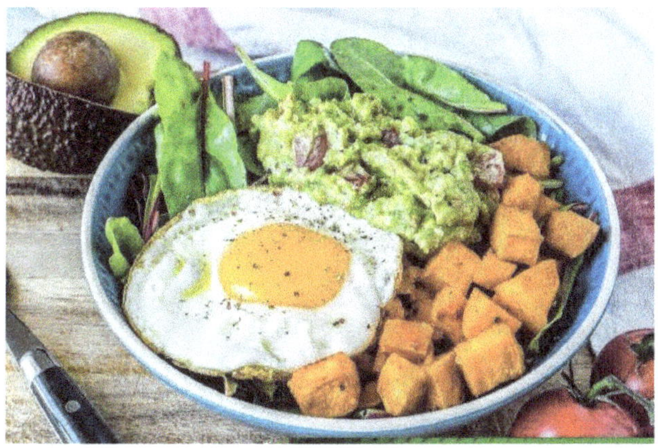

Ingredients:

- Peel and cube one medium-sized sweet potato

- 1 ripe avocado, sliced

- 2 eggs

- 1 tablespoon olive oil

- Salt and pepper to taste

- 1 teaspoon paprika

- 1/4 cup feta cheese, crumbled

- Fresh cilantro or parsley for garnish

Procedure:

- Preheat the oven to 400°F (200°C).

- Toss sweet potato cubes in olive oil, salt, pepper, and paprika. Spread them on a baking sheet and roast for 20-25 minutes or until tender.
- While sweet potatoes are roasting, poach or fry the eggs to your liking.
- In a serving bowl, arrange the roasted sweet potatoes, sliced avocado, and eggs.
- Sprinkle with crumbled feta cheese and garnish with fresh cilantro or parsley.

Time of Preparation:

- Approximately 30-35 minutes.

Tips and Tricks:

- Customize by adding cherry tomatoes, spinach, or a drizzle of hot sauce for extra flavor.
- Opt for poached eggs for a runny yolk that blends deliciously with the sweet potato and avocado.
- Prepping sweet potatoes in advance can save time during busy mornings.

Nutritional Value per Serving:

- Calories: Approximately 400-450 kcal
- Protein: 15g
- Healthy Fats: 25g
- Carbohydrates: 35g
- Dietary Fiber: 9g

Health Benefits:

- Sweet potatoes are rich in vitamins A and C, providing immune support.
- Avocado offers healthy monounsaturated fats and additional vitamins.
- Eggs contribute high-quality protein and essential nutrients.
- Feta cheese provides calcium and a burst of flavor.
- Olive oil adds heart-healthy monounsaturated fats.

- Keep an eye on portion sizes, especially if you are monitoring calorie intake.

- Adjust salt levels based on personal dietary needs.

- If allergic to any ingredients, omit or substitute accordingly.

Chia Seed Pudding Parfait

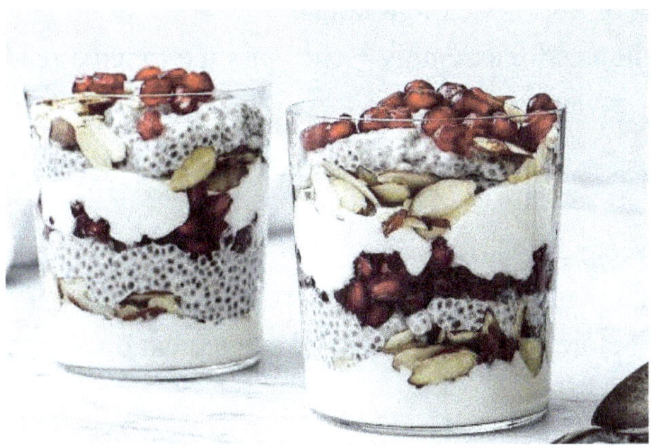

Ingredients:

For Chia Seed Pudding:

- 1/4 cup chia seeds
- 1 cup almond milk (or any milk of choice)
- 1 tablespoon maple syrup or honey
- 1/2 teaspoon vanilla extract

For Parfait Layers:

- Greek yogurt
- Fresh berries (strawberries, blueberries, raspberries)
- Granola
- Sliced bananas
- Honey for drizzling

For Chia Seed Pudding:

- Combine almond milk, vanilla essence, maple syrup (or honey), and chia seeds in a bowl.
- Cover and refrigerate for at least 3 hours or overnight, allowing the chia seeds to absorb the liquid and form a pudding-like consistency.

Assembly:

- In serving glasses or bowls, layer chia seed pudding, Greek yogurt, fresh berries, granola, and sliced bananas.
- Continue layering until you reach the top, then sprinkle some honey on top.
- Optionally, garnish with additional berries or a sprinkle of granola.
- Time of Preparation: Approximately 10 minutes for assembly + chilling time for chia seed pudding.

Tips and Tricks:

- Experiment with different fruits, nuts, or seeds for variety.
- Use flavored yogurt or add a touch of cinnamon to enhance the layers.
- Preparing the chia seed pudding the night before ensures a quick and convenient breakfast.

Nutritional Value per Serving:

- Calories: Approximately 300-350 kcal
- Protein: 10g
- Healthy Fats: 12g
- Carbohydrates: 40g
- Dietary Fiber: 12g

Health Benefits:

- Chia seeds are rich in omega-3 fatty acids and provide a good source of fiber.
- Greek yogurt adds probiotics for gut health and protein.
- Berries are loaded with antioxidants and vitamins.
- Almond milk contributes to the overall creaminess with fewer calories compared to dairy milk.

Caution:

- Monitor portion sizes if you are mindful of calorie intake.
- Adjust sweetness levels based on personal preference.

- Individuals with nut allergies should choose a milk alternative accordingly.

3

Lunch Bowls

Mediterranean Chickpea Salad Bowl

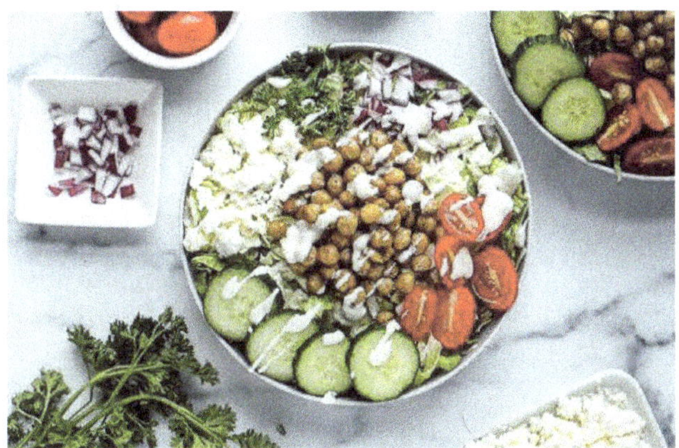

Ingredients:

- 1 can (15 oz) chickpeas, drained and rinsed
- 1 cup cherry tomatoes, halved
- 1 cucumber, diced
- 1/2 red onion, finely chopped
- 1/2 cup Kalamata olives, pitted and sliced
- 1/2 cup feta cheese, crumbled
- 1/4 cup fresh parsley, chopped
- 1/4 cup extra virgin olive oil
- 2 tablespoons red wine vinegar
- 1 teaspoon dried oregano
- Salt and pepper to taste

Procedure:

- Prepare Chickpeas: In a skillet over medium heat, sauté chickpeas with a drizzle of olive oil until golden brown. Season with salt and pepper. Set aside to cool.
- Combine Vegetables: In a large bowl, mix cherry tomatoes, cucumber, red onion, olives, and cooled chickpeas.

- Make Dressing: In a small bowl, whisk together olive oil, red wine vinegar, dried oregano, salt, and pepper. Adjust seasoning to taste.
- Assemble Salad: Pour the dressing over the vegetable mixture and toss gently to coat evenly. Sprinkle feta cheese and fresh parsley on top.
- Serve: Divide the salad into bowls and serve immediately, or refrigerate for a couple of hours to let flavors meld.

Time of Preparation:

- Approximately 15-20 minutes.

Tips and Tricks:

- For an extra burst of flavor, marinate the salad in the refrigerator for a few hours before serving.
- Customize with additional ingredients like roasted red peppers or artichoke hearts.
- Use fresh, high-quality ingredients for the best taste.

Nutritional Value per Serving:

- Calories: ~350 kcal
- Protein: ~10g
- Fat: ~20g
- Carbohydrates: ~30g
- Fiber: ~8g

Health Benefits:

- Rich in fiber and plant-based protein from chickpeas, promoting digestive health and satiety.
- Olive oil provides heart-healthy monounsaturated fats.
- Abundance of antioxidants from tomatoes, olives, and parsley.

- Watch portion sizes, especially if aiming for a lower-calorie intake.
- Be mindful of sodium content, especially in feta cheese and olives for those with dietary restrictions.

Thai Peanut Tofu Bowl

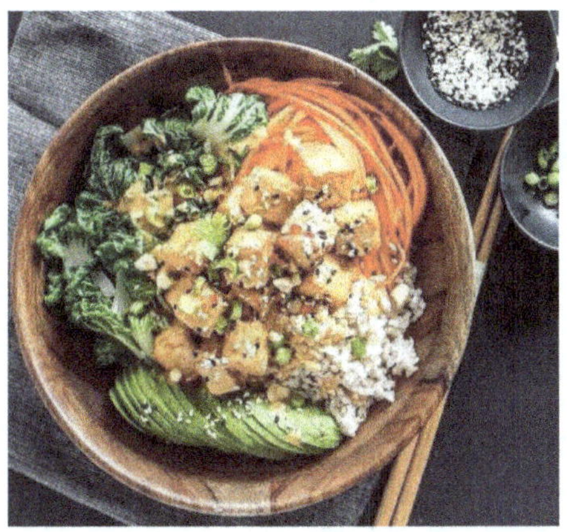

Ingredients:

For Tofu:

- 1 block (14 oz) extra-firm tofu, pressed and cubed
- 2 tablespoons soy sauce
- 1 tablespoon sesame oil
- 1 tablespoon cornstarch

For Bowl:

- 1 cup cooked quinoa or brown rice
- 1 cup shredded red cabbage
- 1 bell pepper, thinly sliced

- 1 carrot, julienned
- 1/2 cup edamame, shelled
- 2 green onions, chopped
- Sesame seeds for garnish

For Peanut Sauce:

- 1/4 cup peanut butter
- 2 tablespoons soy sauce
- 1 tablespoon rice vinegar
- 1 tablespoon maple syrup
- 1 clove garlic, minced
- 1 teaspoon grated ginger
- Water to thin, if needed

Procedure:

- Prepare Tofu: In a bowl, mix soy sauce, sesame oil, and cornstarch Coat the tofu cubes by tossing them in the mixture. Bake or pan-fry until crispy.
- Make Peanut Sauce: Whisk together peanut butter, soy sauce, rice vinegar, maple syrup, garlic, and ginger. Adjust consistency with water to reach desired thickness.
- Assemble Bowl: Arrange cooked quinoa or brown rice in bowls. Top with shredded cabbage, bell pepper, julienned carrot, edamame, and crispy tofu.
- Drizzle with Peanut Sauce: Pour peanut sauce generously over the bowl.
- Add sesame seeds and chopped green onions as garnish.
- Serve: Toss the bowl ingredients together before eating to distribute the flavors evenly.

Time of Preparation:

- Approximately 30 minutes.

- For extra flavor, marinate tofu in soy sauce and sesame oil for 30 minutes before coating in cornstarch.
- Adjust the spice level of the peanut sauce with red pepper flakes or sriracha.
- Customize veggies based on personal preferences.

Nutritional Value per Serving:

- Calories: ~500 kcal
- Protein: ~20g
- Fat: ~25g
- Carbohydrates: ~50g
- Fiber: ~10g

Health Benefits:

- Tofu provides plant-based protein.
- Vitamins, minerals, and antioxidants that are necessary are found in vegetables.
- Peanut sauce contains healthy fats and protein.

Caution:

- Watch portion sizes for those on calorie-restricted diets.
- Check peanut butter ingredients for added sugars or unhealthy fats.

Roasted Vegetable and Hummus Quinoa Bowl

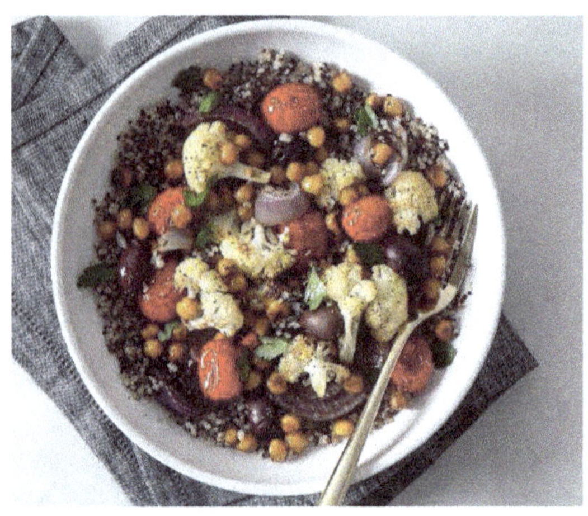

Ingredients:

For Roasted Vegetables:

- 1 zucchini, sliced
- 1 bell pepper, cut into strips
- 1 cup cherry tomatoes, halved
- 1 red onion, sliced
- 2 tablespoons olive oil
- 1 teaspoon dried thyme
- Salt and pepper to taste

For Quinoa:

- 1 cup quinoa, rinsed
- 2 cups vegetable broth or water
- For Assembly:
- 1 cup hummus
- 1/4 cup fresh parsley, chopped
- 1/4 cup feta cheese, crumbled
- Lemon wedges for serving

- Preheat Oven: Preheat the oven to 400°F (200°C).
- Roast Vegetables: Toss zucchini, bell pepper, cherry tomatoes, and red onion in olive oil, dried thyme, salt, and pepper. Spread on a baking sheet and roast for 20-25 minutes or until vegetables are tender and slightly caramelized.
- To cook quinoa, put it in a saucepan with water or vegetable broth. Bring to a boil, then reduce heat, cover, and simmer for 15 minutes or until quinoa is cooked and liquid is absorbed. Fluff with a fork.
- Assemble Bowl: In each bowl, layer cooked quinoa, roasted vegetables, and a generous dollop of hummus.
- Garnish: Sprinkle fresh parsley and crumbled feta cheese on top.
- Serve: Squeeze lemon wedges over the bowl before serving for added freshness.

Time of Preparation:

- Approximately 45 minutes.

Tips and Tricks:

- Try a variety of veggies depending on what's in season.
- Drizzle a bit of balsamic glaze over the roasted vegetables for extra flavor.
- Use flavored hummus for a unique twist.

Nutritional Value per Serving:

- Calories: ~450 kcal
- Protein: ~15g
- Fat: ~20g
- Carbohydrates: ~55g
- Fiber: ~10g

Health Benefits:

- Quinoa provides a complete protein source.
- Roasted vegetables offer a variety of vitamins, minerals, and antioxidants.
- Hummus adds healthy fats and additional protein.

Caution:

- Be mindful of portion sizes for those on specific dietary plans.
- Check hummus ingredients for added sugars or unhealthy additives.

4

Dinner Bowls

Spicy Black Bean and Corn Bowl

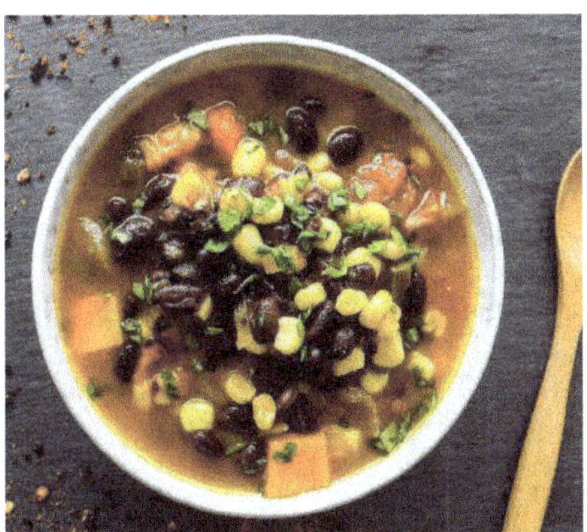

- One cup of washed, drained, and cooked black beans (from can).
- One cup frozen or fresh corn kernels1 cup cherry tomatoes, halved
- 1 avocado, diced
- 1/2 red onion, finely chopped
- 1 jalapeño pepper, finely diced
- 1/4 cup fresh cilantro, chopped
- 1 lime, juiced
- 2 tablespoons olive oil
- 1 teaspoon ground cumin
- 1 teaspoon chili powder
- Salt and pepper to taste
- 2 cups cooked brown rice or quinoa

Procedures:

Prepare the Base:

- Cook brown rice or quinoa according to package instructions.

Sauté Vegetables:

- In a large skillet, heat olive oil over medium heat.
- Sauté red onion, jalapeño, and corn until are tender.
- Heat the olive oil in a big skillet over medium heat.
- Sauté the corn, jalapeño, and red onion until the veggies are soft.

- Add the beans and season vegetables
- Add chili powder, black beans, ground cumin, salt, and pepper.
- Simmer the beans until they are thoroughly heated.

Put the Bowl Together:

- Arrange cooked rice or quinoa in layers in serving bowls.
- Top with the spicy black bean mixture.

Add Fresh Elements:

- Arrange cherry tomatoes, diced avocado, and chopped cilantro on top.

Finish with Lime Juice:

- Pour some lime juice into the bowl to give it a zesty boost.

Time of Preparation:

- Approximately 30 minutes.

Tips and Tricks:

- Customize spice level by adjusting jalapeño quantity.
- Enhance flavor with a drizzle of hot sauce or a sprinkle of smoked paprika.
- Prepare extra and store in airtight containers for quick, healthy lunches.

Nutritional Value per Serving:

- Calories: ~400 kcal
- Protein: ~10g
- Fiber: ~12g
- Healthy Fats: ~15g
- Vitamins and Minerals: Rich in vitamin C, potassium, and folate.

Health Benefits:

- High fiber content promotes digestive health.
- Plant-based proteins from beans and grains support muscle health.
- Avocado provides heart-healthy monounsaturated fats.

Caution:

- Be mindful of spice levels, especially if sensitive to heat.

- Pay attention to portion sizes to reduce calorie intake.

Teriyaki Glazed Tempeh Bowl

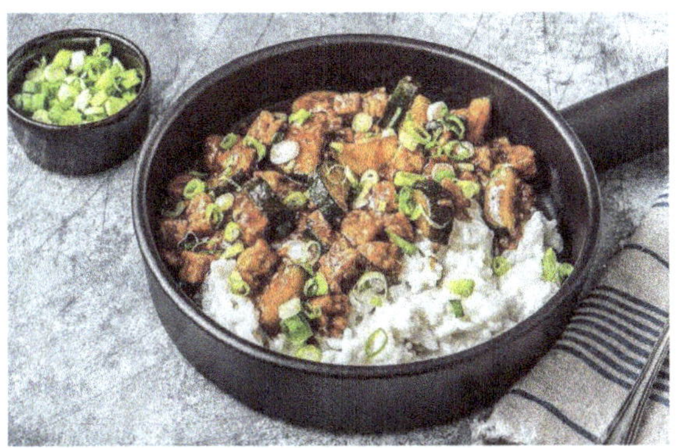

Ingredients:

- 1 package (about 8 oz) tempeh, sliced into thin strips
- 1 cup broccoli florets
- 1 carrot, julienned
- 1 red bell pepper, sliced
- 2 cups cooked brown rice or quinoa
- Two thinly sliced green onions (for garnish)
- Sesame seeds (for garnish)

For Teriyaki Glaze:

- 1/4 cup soy sauce
- 2 tablespoons mirin
- 2 tablespoons rice vinegar
- 2 tablespoons maple syrup or honey
- 1 teaspoon grated ginger
- 1 clove garlic, minced

- To thicken, combine 1 tablespoon cornstarch with 2 tablespoons water.

Procedures:

Prepare Tempeh:

- Steam tempeh for about 10 minutes to reduce bitterness.

- Slice into thin strips.

Sauté Vegetables:

- In a pan, stir-fry broccoli, carrot, and red bell pepper until slightly tender.

Cook Tempeh:

- In the same pan, add tempeh strips and cook until golden brown.

Prepare Teriyaki Glaze:

- In a bowl, mix soy sauce, mirin, rice vinegar, maple syrup, grated ginger, and minced garlic.
- Pour the mixture into the pan with tempeh and vegetables.

Thicken the Sauce:

- Pour the cornstarch mixture into the pan and stir until the sauce thickens.

Assemble the Bowl:

- In serving bowls, layer cooked rice or quinoa.
- Top with teriyaki-glazed tempeh and sautéed vegetables.

Garnish:

- Sprinkle sliced green onions and sesame seeds on top.

Time of Preparation:

- Approximately 45 minutes.

Tips and Tricks:

- Marinate tempeh in teriyaki sauce for extra flavor.
- For an extra spicy kick, add a sprinkle of red pepper flakes.
- Try different vegetables like snap peas or mushrooms for variety.

Nutritional Value per Serving:

- Calories: ~450 kcal
- Protein: ~20g
- Fiber: ~10g
- Healthy Fats: ~15g
- Rich in iron, calcium, and vitamin C.

- Tempeh provides plant-based protein and probiotics.
- A multitude of vitamins and antioxidants can be found in vegetables.
- Teriyaki glaze is lower in sodium compared to store-bought versions.

Caution:

- Monitor sodium intake, especially for those with hypertension.
- Check tempeh for allergies; it contains soy.

Cauliflower and Chickpea Curry Bowl

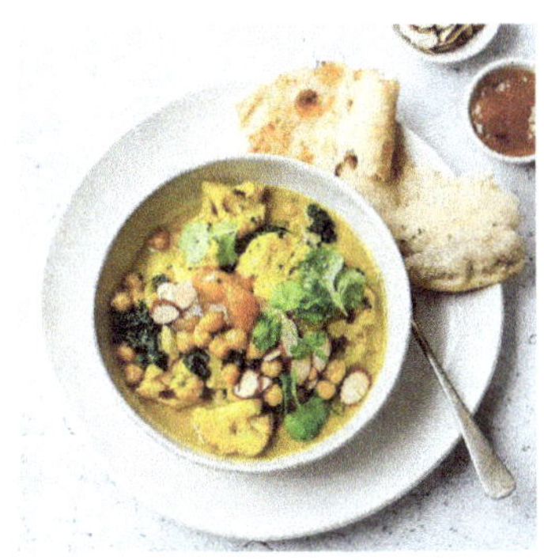

Ingredients:

- 1 medium cauliflower, cut into florets
- 1 can (15 oz) chickpeas, drained and rinsed
- 1 onion, finely chopped
- 3 cloves garlic, minced
- 1 tablespoon ginger, grated
- 1 can (14 oz) diced tomatoes
- 1 can (14 oz) coconut milk
- 2 tablespoons curry powder
- 1 teaspoon ground cumin
- 1 teaspoon ground coriander
- 1/2 teaspoon turmeric

- 1/4 teaspoon cayenne pepper (optional for extra heat)
- Salt and pepper to taste
- 2 tablespoons cooking oil
- Fresh cilantro, chopped (for garnish)
- Cooked basmati rice or quinoa (for serving)

Procedures:

Sauté Aromatics:

- Heat the oil in a big pot over medium heat.
- Add chopped onion, minced garlic, and grated ginger. Sauté until softened.

Spice it Up:

- Stir in curry powder, ground cumin, ground coriander, turmeric, and cayenne pepper (if using).
- Cook for a minute until fragrant.

Add Cauliflower and Chickpeas:

- Add cauliflower florets and chickpeas to the pot.

- Stir to distribute the fragrant spices.

Pour in Tomatoes and Coconut Milk:

- Add diced tomatoes and coconut milk to the pot.
- Season with salt and pepper.
- Bring to a simmer and let it cook until cauliflower is tender.

Simmer to Perfection:

- Simmer the curry for about 20-25 minutes, allowing the flavors to meld.

Adjust Seasoning:

- Taste and adjust salt and pepper as needed.
- Add more spice if desired.

Serve:

- Spoon the curry over cooked basmati rice or quinoa.

Garnish and Enjoy:

- Garnish with fresh cilantro before serving.

- Approximately 45 minutes.

- Add a squeeze of lime or lemon juice at the end for a burst of freshness.
- Customize the spice level by adjusting cayenne pepper or adding chili flakes.
- Experiment with different vegetables like spinach or sweet potatoes.

- Calories: ~350 kcal
- Protein: ~10g
- Fiber: ~10g
- Healthy Fats: ~20g
- Excellent source of vitamin C, fiber, and plant-based protein.

- Cauliflower provides antioxidants and is rich in vitamins.
- Chickpeas provide an increase in fiber and protein.
- Coconut milk adds healthy fats and a creamy texture.

- Be mindful of portion sizes to control calorie intake.
- Monitor spice levels, especially for those sensitive to heat.

5

Protein-Packed Bowls

Lentil and Spinach Power Bowl

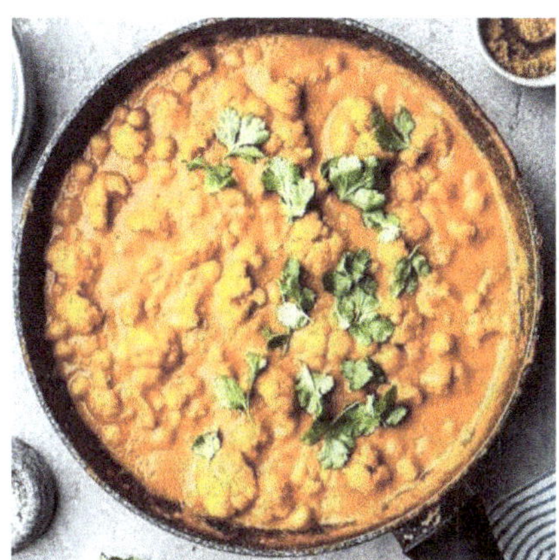

Ingredients:

- 1 cup green lentils, rinsed
- 2 cups fresh spinach, chopped
- 1 cup cherry tomatoes, halved
- 1 cucumber, diced
- 1 red bell pepper, sliced
- 1/4 cup red onion, finely chopped
- 1/3 cup feta cheese, crumbled
- 1/4 cup extra-virgin olive oil
- 2 tablespoons balsamic vinegar
- 1 teaspoon Dijon mustard
- 1 clove garlic, minced
- Salt and pepper to taste
- 1 teaspoon dried oregano

Procedures:

- Cook lentils according to package instructions; typically, simmer in water for 20-25 minutes until tender but not mushy. Drain any excess water.
- In a large bowl, combine cooked lentils, spinach, cherry tomatoes, cucumber, red bell pepper, red onion, and feta cheese.
- In a small bowl, whisk together olive oil, balsamic vinegar, Dijon mustard, minced garlic, salt, pepper, and dried oregano to create the dressing.
- Pour the dressing over the lentil and vegetable mixture. Toss gently until well-coated.

- Allow the bowl to marinate for at least 15 minutes before serving to enhance flavors.

Time of Preparation:

- Approximately 30 minutes.

Tips and Tricks:

- Customize with additional vegetables or protein sources for variety.
- Drizzle the dressing just before serving to maintain the freshness of the salad.
- Make extra dressing and store it separately for a quick refresh if the salad is stored for later consumption.

Nutritional Value per Serving:

- Calories: 350
- Protein: 18g
- Fiber: 12g
- Healthy Fats: 14g
- Vitamins and Minerals: Rich in iron, vitamin C, and folate.

Health Benefits:

- High fiber content supports digestive health.
- Lentils provide plant-based protein and iron.
- Spinach is a nutrient powerhouse, offering vitamins A, C, and K.
- Olive oil contributes heart-healthy monounsaturated fats.
- Feta cheese adds calcium for bone health.

Caution:

- Individuals with kidney issues may need to moderate lentil intake due to their purine content.
- Adjust salt intake based on dietary requirements.

Edamame and Brown Rice Bowl

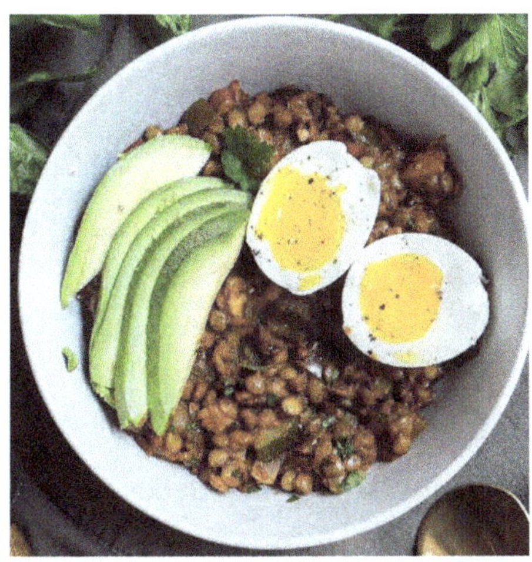

Ingredients:

- 1 cup brown rice, uncooked
- 2 cups edamame, shelled
- 1 carrot, julienned
- 1 red bell pepper, thinly sliced
- 1/4 cup green onions, chopped
- 2 tablespoons sesame seeds, toasted
- 2 tablespoons soy sauce (low sodium)
- 1 tablespoon rice vinegar
- 1 tablespoon sesame oil
- 1 teaspoon ginger, grated
- 1 clove garlic, minced
- 1 teaspoon honey
- Salt and pepper to taste

Procedures:

- Cook brown rice according to package instructions, typically simmering for 45-50 minutes. Fluff with a fork and let it cool.
- In a pot of boiling water, blanch edamame for 3-5 minutes or until tender. Drain and set aside.
- In a large bowl, combine cooked brown rice, edamame, julienned carrot, sliced red bell pepper, green onions, and toasted sesame seeds.

- In a small bowl, whisk together soy sauce, rice vinegar, sesame oil, grated ginger, minced garlic, honey, salt, and pepper to create the dressing.
- Drizzle the rice and veggie combination with the dressing. Toss gently until everything is well-coated.
- Let the bowl sit for 10 minutes to allow flavors to meld before serving.

Time of Preparation:

- Approximately 60 minutes.

Tips and Tricks:

- Use pre-cooked or frozen brown rice for a quicker meal.
- Customize with your favorite vegetables like broccoli or snow peas.
- Experiment with different toppings like sliced avocado or a sprinkle of nori flakes.

Nutritional Value per Serving:

- Calories: 400
- Protein: 15g
- Fiber: 10g
- Healthy Fats: 12g
- Vitamins and Minerals: High in manganese, folate, and vitamin K.

Health Benefits:

- Complex carbs included in brown rice provide you energy for the long term.
- Edamame is a great plant-based source of fiber and protein.
- Sesame seeds provide necessary nutrients and good lipids.
- A range of vitamins and antioxidants can be found in vegetables.

Caution:

- Monitor soy sauce intake for those watching sodium levels.
- Adjust honey or sugar based on personal dietary preferences.

Walnut and Cranberry Quinoa Bowl

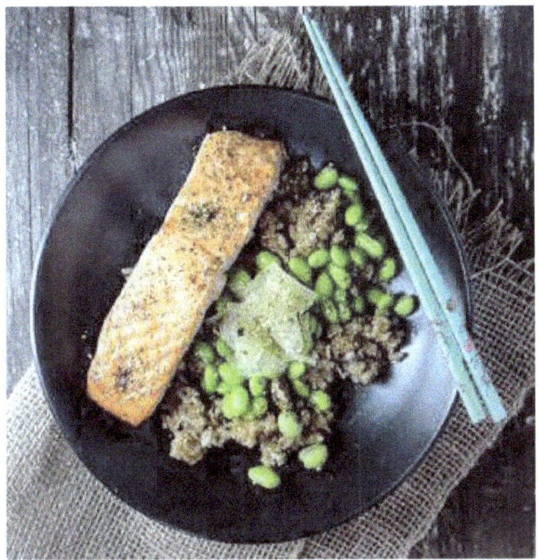

- 1 cup quinoa, rinsed
- 2 cups water or vegetable broth
- 1/2 cup walnuts, chopped and toasted
- 1/2 cup dried cranberries
- 1 cup baby spinach, chopped
- 1/4 cup red onion, finely diced
- 1/4 cup feta cheese, crumbled
- 2 tablespoons olive oil
- 1 tablespoon balsamic vinegar
- 1 teaspoon maple syrup
- Salt and pepper to taste
- Fresh parsley for garnish (optional)

Procedures:

- Put the quinoa and water or vegetable broth in a medium-sized saucepan. Bring to a boil, then reduce heat, cover, and simmer for 15-20 minutes until quinoa is cooked and water is absorbed.
- Fluff quinoa with a fork and let it cool to room temperature.
- In a dry skillet over medium heat, toast chopped walnuts until golden and fragrant, stirring frequently.

- In a large bowl, combine cooked quinoa, toasted walnuts, dried cranberries, chopped spinach, diced red onion, and crumbled feta cheese.
- In a small bowl, whisk together olive oil, balsamic vinegar, maple syrup, salt, and pepper to create the dressing.
- Drizzle the quinoa mixture with the dressing, then gently toss to blend.
- Garnish with fresh parsley if desired.

Time of Preparation:

- Approximately 30 minutes.

Tips and Tricks:

- Cook quinoa in vegetable broth for added flavor.
- Customize with additional veggies like cherry tomatoes or cucumbers.
- Adjust sweetness by modifying the amount of maple syrup in the dressing.

Nutritional Value per Serving:

- Calories: 380
- Protein: 10g
- Fiber: 7g
- Healthy Fats: 18g
- Vitamins and Minerals: Rich in omega-3 fatty acids, vitamin E, and iron.

Health Benefits:

- Quinoa is a complete protein and an excellent source of vital amino acids.
- Walnuts offer heart-healthy omega-3 fatty acids.
- Cranberries add antioxidants and vitamin C.
- Spinach contributes iron and vitamin K.

Caution:

- Watch portion sizes as nuts and dried fruits can be calorie-dense.
- Check cranberry packaging for added sugars.

6

Quick and Easy Bowls

15-Minute Avocado and Black Bean Bowl

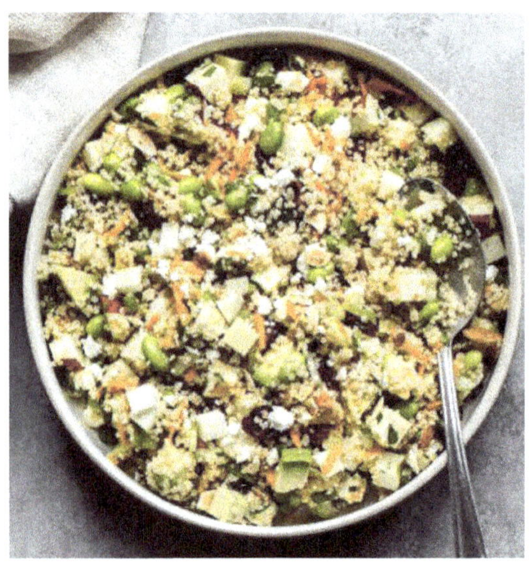

- 1 ripe avocado, diced
- 1 can (15 oz) black beans, drained and rinsed
- 1 cup cherry tomatoes, halved
- 1/2 cup red onion, finely chopped
- 1/4 cup fresh cilantro, chopped
- 1 lime, juiced
- 2 tablespoons olive oil
- 1 teaspoon cumin
- Salt and pepper to taste
- Optional toppings: shredded cheese, Greek yogurt, salsa

Procedures:

- Heat the olive oil in a big skillet over medium-high heat.

- Place the sliced almonds and minced garlic in the skillet and cook until the almonds are golden brown.

- When the broccoli florets are crisp-tender, add them to the skillet and stir-fry for three to four minutes.

- Combine the sesame oil, honey, and soy sauce in a small bowl. After adding the mixture, toss the broccoli and almonds to ensure even coating.

- Simmer for a further two to three minutes to let the flavors combine.

- Serve the broccoli and almond combination over cooked rice or quinoa, if desired. Sprinkle sesame seeds on top for flavor and texture.

Time of Preparation:

- 15 minutes

Tips and Tricks:

- Choose ripe avocados for creaminess.
- Customize with additional veggies like corn or bell peppers.

- Try a variety of toppings to find what suits your palate best.

Nutritional Value per Serving:

- Calories: Approximately 300-350 calories
- Protein: 10-15g
- Fiber: 12-15g
- Healthy fats from avocado and olive oil

Health Benefits:

- Rich in fiber for digestive health.
- Avocado provides heart-healthy monounsaturated fats.
- Black beans offer plant-based protein and essential minerals.

Caution:

- Be mindful of portion sizes for calorie control.
- If allergic to any ingredients, substitute accordingly.
- Individuals with kidney issues may want to monitor potassium intake due to avocado content.

Speedy Broccoli and Almond Bowl

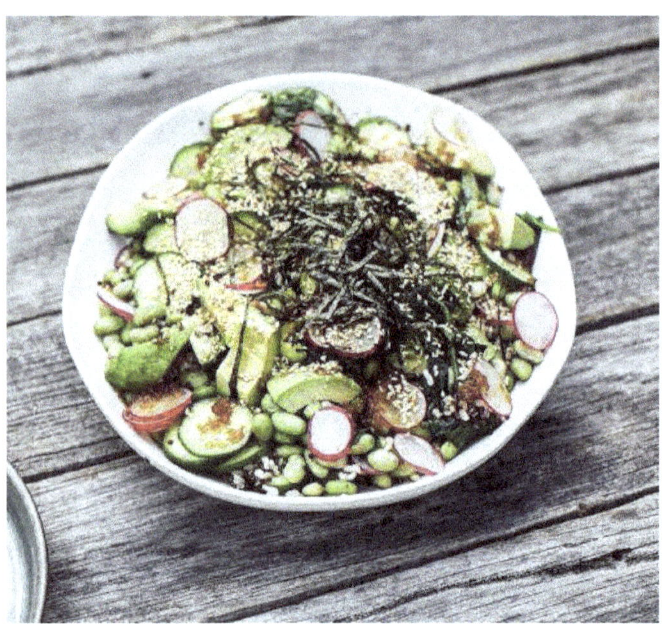

- 2 cups broccoli florets
- 1/2 cup sliced almonds
- 2 cloves garlic, minced
- 2 tablespoons olive oil
- 1 tablespoon soy sauce
- 1 teaspoon honey
- 1 teaspoon sesame oil
- Sesame seeds for garnish (optional)
- Cooked quinoa or rice (optional, for serving)

Procedures:

- In a large skillet, heat olive oil over medium-high heat.
- Add minced garlic and sliced almonds to the skillet, sautéing until the almonds turn golden brown.

- Add broccoli florets to the skillet and stir-fry for 3-4 minutes until they are crisp-tender.
- In a small bowl, whisk together soy sauce, honey, and sesame oil. Pour the mixture over the broccoli and almonds, tossing to coat evenly.
- Cook for an additional 2-3 minutes, allowing the flavors to meld.
- Optional: Serve the broccoli and almond mixture over cooked quinoa or rice.
- Garnish with sesame seeds for added texture and flavor.

Time of Preparation:

- 15 minutes

Tips and Tricks:

- Use pre-cut broccoli florets for a quicker preparation.
- Toast almonds before adding broccoli for enhanced nutty flavor.
- Adjust honey and soy sauce quantities to suit your taste preferences.
- Nutritional Value per Serving:
- Calories: Approximately 250-300 calories
- Protein: 8-10g
- Healthy fats from almonds and olive oil
- Low in saturated fat

Health Benefits:

- Broccoli provides vitamins C and K, fiber, and antioxidants.
- Almonds offer healthy fats, protein, and vitamin E.
- The dish is a good source of plant-based nutrients and can be part of a balanced diet.

Caution:

- If allergic to any ingredients, substitute accordingly.
- Be cautious with portion sizes, especially if combining with rice or quinoa for calorie control.
- Individuals with nut allergies should omit almonds or choose an alternative.

Instant Pot Lentil and Vegetable Bowl

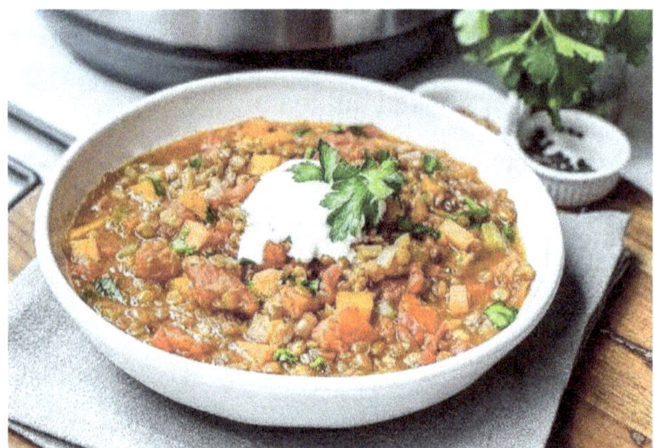

Ingredients:

- One cup of washed and drained dried brown lentils
- 1 onion, finely chopped
- 2 carrots, diced
- 2 celery stalks, chopped
- 1 bell pepper, diced
- 3 cloves garlic, minced
- 1 can (14 oz) diced tomatoes
- 4 cups vegetable broth
- 1 teaspoon ground cumin
- 1 teaspoon smoked paprika
- 1/2 teaspoon turmeric
- Salt and pepper to taste
- 2 cups spinach or kale, chopped
- 2 tablespoons olive oil
- Lemon wedges for serving

- Set Instant Pot to sauté mode and heat olive oil. Add the bell pepper, celery, carrots, and onion, chopped. Sauté until vegetables are softened.
- Add minced garlic, ground cumin, smoked paprika, turmeric, salt, and pepper. Stir to combine.
- Add dry brown lentils, diced tomatoes, and vegetable broth to the Instant Pot. Stir well.
- Cancel sauté mode, secure the lid, and set the Instant Pot to manual high pressure for 15 minutes.
- Once cooking is complete, allow for a natural pressure release for 5 minutes, then quick release any remaining pressure.
- Stir in chopped spinach or kale, allowing it to wilt in the residual heat.
- Adjust seasoning if necessary and serve hot. Squeeze fresh lemon juice over each serving for brightness.

Time of Preparation:

- Approximately 30 minutes (including Instant Pot time)

Tips and Tricks:

- Use green or brown lentils for better texture.
- Customize with additional vegetables like zucchini or sweet potatoes.
- Experiment with spices to suit your taste preferences.

Nutritional Value per Serving:

- Calories: Approximately 300-350 calories
- Protein: 15-18g
- High in fiber, vitamins, and minerals
- Low in saturated fat

Health Benefits:

- Plant-based fiber and protein can be found in abundance in lentils.

- Abundant vegetables provide essential vitamins and antioxidants.

- The dish is low in fat and cholesterol, supporting heart health.

- If using pre-seasoned broth, adjust salt accordingly.

- Monitor lentil cooking times, as older lentils may take longer.

- Individuals with specific dietary restrictions or allergies should check ingredients for suitability.

Fresh Spring Asparagus and Pea Bowl

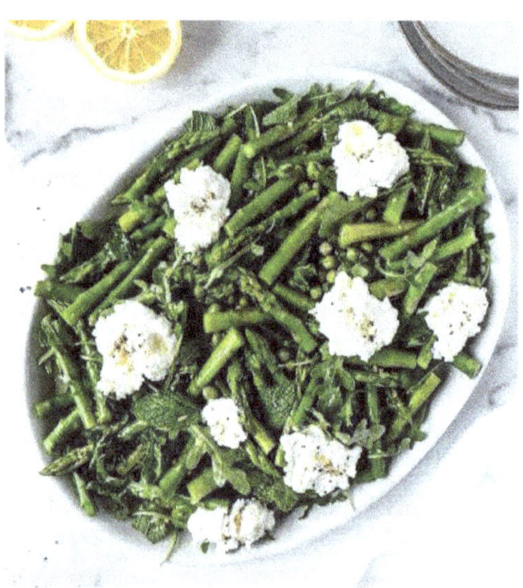

Ingredients:

- 1 bunch fresh asparagus, trimmed
- 1 cup fresh or frozen peas
- 1 cup quinoa, rinsed
- 1 lemon, juiced
- 2 tablespoons olive oil
- 2 cloves garlic, minced

- Salt and pepper to taste
- 1/4 cup chopped fresh mint
- 1/4 cup crumbled feta cheese (optional)

- To prepare the quinoa, put two cups of water and the quinoa in a saucepan. Bring to a boil, then reduce heat, cover, and simmer for 15-20 minutes or until quinoa is cooked and water is absorbed.
- Blanch Asparagus and Peas: While quinoa is cooking, bring a pot of water to boil. Add asparagus and peas, cook for 2-3 minutes until just tender. Quickly transfer them to an ice water bath to preserve their vibrant color.
- Make Dressing: In a small bowl, whisk together olive oil, lemon juice, minced garlic, salt, and pepper. Adjust the seasoning to taste.
- Assemble Bowl: Fluff the cooked quinoa with a fork and divide it among serving bowls. Arrange blanched asparagus and peas on top Over the quinoa and vegetables, drizzle the dressing.
- Garnish and Serve: Sprinkle chopped mint and crumbled feta (if using) over the bowls. Serve immediately, allowing the flavors to meld.

Time of Preparation:

- Approximately 30-40 minutes.

Tips and Tricks:

- • Break off the tough ends of the asparagus to trim it. They naturally break where the tender part begins.
- For added flavor, toast the quinoa in a dry pan before boiling.

Nutritional Value per Serving:

- Calories: 350-400
- Protein: 12g
- Fiber: 8g
- Healthy fats: 14g
- Vitamin C: 40% of daily recommended intake

Health Benefits:

- Asparagus is rich in vitamins A, C, and K, as well as folate.
- Peas provide plant-based protein, fiber, and essential nutrients like vitamin K.

- Quinoa is a complete protein source, offering all essential amino acids.
- Olive oil contributes heart-healthy monounsaturated fats.

- Those with kidney issues should monitor asparagus intake due to its oxalate content.
- Individuals allergic to peas or quinoa should choose alternative ingredients.
- Adjust portion sizes based on dietary needs and calorie goals.

Summer Harvest Grain Bowl

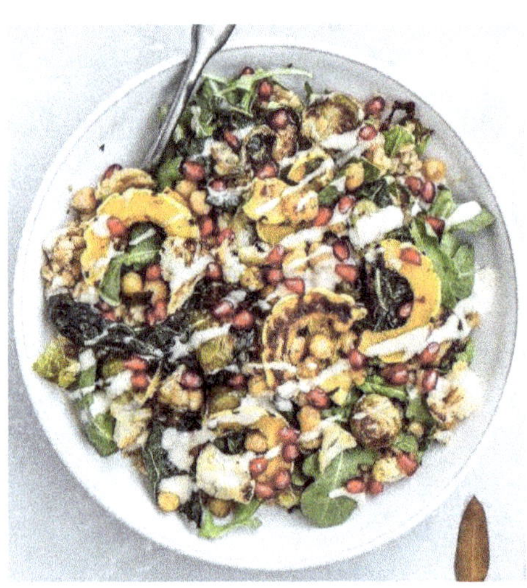

Ingredients:

- 1 cup cooked quinoa
- 1 cup cooked farro
- 1 cup cherry tomatoes, halved
- 1 cup cucumber, diced
- One cup of fresh or, if frozen, thawed corn kernels
- 1/2 cup red onion, finely chopped
- 1/4 cup fresh basil, chopped
- 1/4 cup feta cheese, crumbled
- 2 tablespoons balsamic vinaigrette
- Salt and pepper to taste
- Grilled chicken or tofu (optional for added protein)

- Prepare Grains: Cook quinoa and farro according to package instructions. Let them cool until they reach room temperature. Combine Ingredients: In a large bowl, mix together cooked quinoa, farro, cherry tomatoes, cucumber, corn, red onion, and fresh basil.
- Add Cheese: Gently fold in the crumbled feta cheese to the grain mixture.
- Dress the Bowl: Drizzle the balsamic vinaigrette over the bowl and toss everything together until well combined. Season with salt and pepper to taste.
- Optional Protein: If desired, top the bowl with grilled chicken or tofu for an extra protein boost.
- Serve: Divide the grain bowl into individual servings and serve immediately.

Time of Preparation:

- Approximately 25-30 minutes.

Tips and Tricks:

- Cook grains ahead of time and store them in the fridge for quicker assembly.
- Experiment with different grains like barley or bulgur for variety.
- Fresh, local produce enhances the flavors; try to source ingredients from a farmers' market if possible.

Nutritional Value per Serving:

- Calories: 400-450
- Protein: 15g
- Fiber: 8g
- Vitamin C: 20% of daily recommended intake
- Calcium: 15% of daily recommended intake

Health Benefits:

- Quinoa and farro provide a mix of complex carbohydrates, fiber, and essential nutrients.
- Tomatoes and basil are rich in antioxidants like lycopene and vitamins A and K.
- Cucumbers contribute hydration and vitamins, while corn adds dietary fiber.

Caution:

- Individuals with gluten sensitivity should choose gluten-free grains.
- Monitor the quantity of cheese for those watching their saturated fat intake.
- Adjust the portion size based on individual dietary needs and goals.

Autumn Pumpkin and Sage Bowl

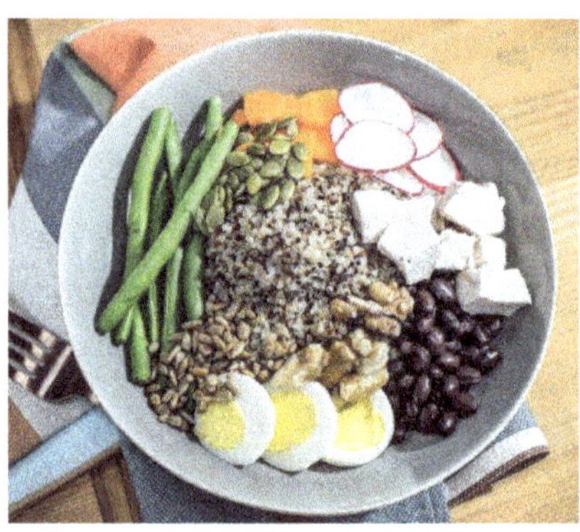

Ingredients:

- 2 cups cubed pumpkin or butternut squash
- 1 cup quinoa, rinsed
- 1 bunch kale, stems removed and leaves torn
- 1/2 cup pecans, chopped
- 1/4 cup dried cranberries
- 2 tablespoons olive oil
- 1 tablespoon maple syrup
- 1 teaspoon ground cinnamon
- 1 teaspoon dried sage
- Salt and pepper to taste
- Goat cheese or feta (optional for garnish)

Procedure:

- Roast Pumpkin: Preheat the oven to 400°F (200°C). Toss pumpkin cubes with olive oil, sage, cinnamon, salt, and pepper. Roast in a single layer on a baking sheet for 20-25 minutes or until tender and slightly caramelized.
- Cook Quinoa: In a saucepan, combine quinoa with 2 cups of water. Bring to a boil, then reduce heat, cover, and simmer for 15-20 minutes or until quinoa is cooked and water is absorbed.
- Massage Kale: In a large bowl, drizzle olive oil over torn kale leaves. Massage the kale for a few minutes to soften it.
- Combine Ingredients: In a serving bowl, layer cooked quinoa, roasted pumpkin, massaged kale, chopped pecans, and dried cranberries.
- Drizzle with Maple Syrup: Drizzle maple syrup over the bowl for a hint of sweetness.

- Optional Garnish: Crumble goat cheese or feta on top for added creaminess (optional).
- Serve: Toss the ingredients together gently and serve warm.

Time of Preparation:

- Approximately 40-45 minutes.

Tips and Tricks:

- Use pre-cut pumpkin to save time or substitute with canned pumpkin puree.
- Toast pecans in a dry pan for a few minutes to enhance their flavor.
- Adjust sweetness by modifying the amount of maple syrup to your liking.

Nutritional Value per Serving:

- Calories: 450-500
- Protein: 12g
- Fiber: 8g
- Vitamin A: 200% of daily recommended intake
- Vitamin C: 30% of daily recommended intake

Health Benefits:

- Beta-carotene, which is abundant in pumpkin, supports eye health.
- Kale provides a powerhouse of vitamins and minerals, including vitamin K and iron.
- Pecans offer healthy fats, fiber, and essential nutrients.
- Cranberries contribute antioxidants and vitamin C.

Caution:

- Monitor portion sizes, especially for those managing carbohydrate intake.
- Those with nut allergies can omit pecans or choose a suitable alternative.
- Adjust seasoning to personal preferences, especially for individuals sensitive to salt.

7

Global Flavors Bowls

Greek-Inspired Mediterranean Bowl

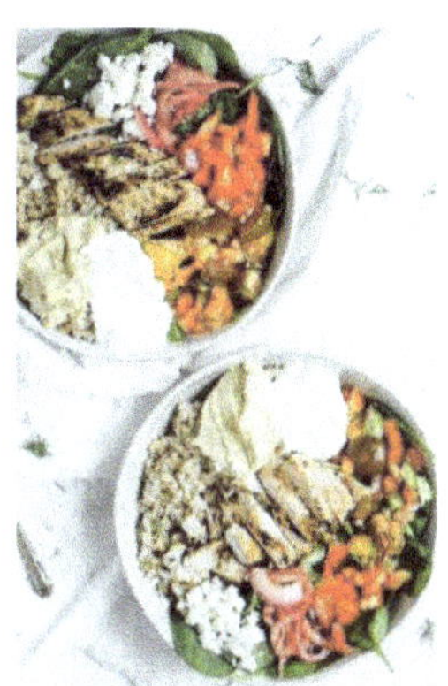

Ingredients:

- For the Base:
- 1 cup quinoa, rinsed
- 2 cups water
- 1 teaspoon olive oil
- Salt to taste

For the Tzatziki Sauce:

- 1 cup Greek yogurt
- 1 cucumber, grated
- 2 cloves garlic, minced
- 1 tablespoon fresh dill, chopped
- 1 tablespoon lemon juice
- Salt and pepper to taste
- For the Grilled Chicken:
- 1 pound chicken breast, boneless and skinless
- 2 tablespoons olive oil
- 1 teaspoon dried oregano
- Salt and pepper to taste
- Lemon wedges for serving

For the Mediterranean Salad:

- 1 cup cherry tomatoes, halved
- 1 cucumber, diced

- 1/2 red onion, finely sliced
- 1/2 cup Kalamata olives, pitted and sliced
- 1/2 cup feta cheese, crumbled
- Fresh parsley, chopped, for garnish

- Cook the Quinoa: In a medium saucepan, combine quinoa, water, olive oil, and salt. Bring to a boil, then reduce heat, cover, and simmer for 15-20 minutes or until quinoa is cooked and water is absorbed.
- Prepare Tzatziki Sauce: In a bowl, mix Greek yogurt, grated cucumber, minced garlic, chopped dill, lemon juice, salt, and pepper. Refrigerate until ready to use.
- Grill the Chicken: Rub chicken breasts with olive oil, dried oregano, salt, and pepper. Cook on the grill for 6 to 8 minutes on each side, or until done. Slice into strips and squeeze lemon juice over the top.
- Assemble the Bowl: Divide cooked quinoa among serving bowls. Top with grilled chicken, cherry tomatoes, diced cucumber, sliced red onion, Kalamata olives, and crumbled feta.
- Drizzle with Tzatziki: Spoon a generous amount of tzatziki sauce over the bowl. Garnish with fresh parsley.

Time of Preparation:

- Approximately 30-40 minutes.

Tips and Tricks:

- Ensure the quinoa is rinsed thoroughly before cooking to remove bitterness.
- Marinate the chicken in olive oil and oregano for enhanced flavor before grilling.

Nutritional Value per Serving:

- Calories: 450-500 kcal
- Protein: 30g
- Carbohydrates: 40g
- Fat: 20g
- Fiber: 6g

Health Benefits:

- High in protein for muscle health.
- Rich in fiber, aiding digestion.
- Abundant in antioxidants from vegetables.

- Heart health benefits from the heart-healthy fats found in olive oil.

- Watch sodium intake, especially if using pre-marinated feta or olives.
- Those with lactose intolerance may consider a lactose-free Greek yogurt for the tzatziki.

Japanese Miso-Ginger Soba Bowl

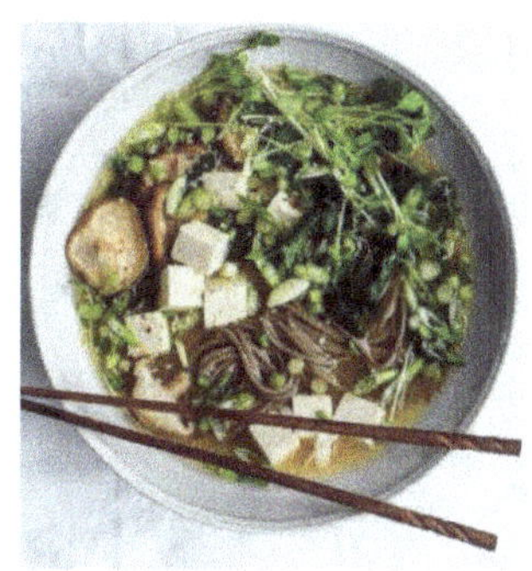

Ingredients:

- For the Soba Noodles:
- 8 oz soba noodles
- 1 tablespoon sesame oil
- 1 tablespoon soy sauce
- For the Miso-Ginger Broth:
- 4 cups vegetable or chicken broth
- 3 tablespoons white miso paste
- 1 tablespoon grated ginger
- 2 cloves garlic, minced
- 2 tablespoons soy sauce
- 1 tablespoon rice vinegar

For the Toppings:

- 1 cup shiitake mushrooms, sliced
- 1 cup spinach, chopped

- 1 carrot, julienned
- 2 green onions, sliced

- As a garnish, add sesame seeds and nori strips.

Procedures:

- Cook Soba Noodles: Cook soba noodles according to package instructions. Drain and toss with sesame oil and soy sauce. Set aside.
- Prepare Miso-Ginger Broth: In a pot, combine broth, white miso paste, grated ginger, minced garlic, soy sauce, and rice vinegar. Bring to a simmer and let it cook for 10-15 minutes to allow flavors to meld.
- Sauté Toppings: In a separate pan, sauté shiitake mushrooms, spinach, and julienned carrots until tender.
- Assemble the Bowl: Divide cooked soba noodles among serving bowls. Ladle miso-ginger broth over the noodles. Top with sautéed vegetables.
- Garnish and Serve: Garnish with sliced green onions, sesame seeds, and nori strips. Serve immediately.

Time of Preparation:

- Approximately 25-30 minutes.

Tips and Tricks:

- Cook soba noodles al dente to prevent them from becoming mushy.
- Adjust miso paste quantity based on personal preference for saltiness.
- Experiment with different vegetable toppings like bok choy or edamame.

Nutritional Value per Serving:

- Calories: 350-400 kcal
- Protein: 12g
- Carbohydrates: 70g
- Fat: 5g
- Fiber: 6g

Health Benefits:

- Soba noodles provide a good source of complex carbohydrates.
- Miso is rich in probiotics and adds beneficial bacteria to the gut.
- Ginger has anti-inflammatory properties, contributing to overall health.

- Be cautious with soy sauce quantity, as it can be high in sodium.
- Those with gluten sensitivity should check soba noodle packaging for wheat content.
- If on a low-sodium diet, opt for a low-sodium broth or reduce soy sauce in the recipe.

Mexican Street Corn Salad Bowl

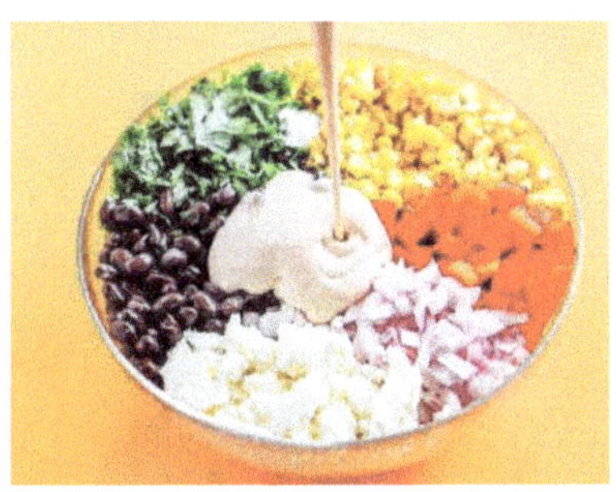

Ingredients:

For the Corn Salad:

- 4 cups corn kernels (fresh or frozen)
- 1 tablespoon olive oil
- 1/2 cup mayonnaise
- 1/2 cup cotija cheese, crumbled
- 1/4 cup fresh cilantro, chopped
- 1 jalapeño, finely chopped (seeds removed for less heat)
- 1 clove garlic, minced
- 1 teaspoon chili powder
- Salt and pepper to taste
- Lime wedges for serving

For the Bowl Base:

- 4 cups cooked rice or quinoa
- 1 can black beans, drained and rinsed
- 1 cup cherry tomatoes, halved

- Avocado slices for garnish

Procedures:

- Roast Corn: If using fresh corn, roast it in a pan with olive oil until slightly charred. If using frozen corn, sauté until heated through.
- Prepare Corn Salad: In a bowl, combine roasted corn, mayonnaise, crumbled cotija cheese, chopped cilantro, jalapeño, minced garlic, chili powder, salt, and pepper. Mix well.
- Assemble the Bowl: Divide cooked rice or quinoa among serving bowls. Top with black beans, cherry tomatoes, and a generous portion of the corn salad.
- Garnish and Serve: Garnish with avocado slices and serve with lime wedges on the side for squeezing over the bowl.

Time of Preparation:

- Approximately 20-25 minutes.

Tips and Tricks:

- Use fresh corn during peak season for optimal flavor.
- Adjust spice level by modifying the amount of jalapeño and chili powder.
- Crumble cotija cheese just before serving for a fresher taste.

Nutritional Value per Serving:

- Calories: 450-500 kcal
- Protein: 10g
- Carbohydrates: 70g
- Fat: 15g
- Fiber: 10g

Health Benefits:

- Corn provides fiber and essential nutrients.
- Black beans provide fiber and plant-based protein.
- Avocado contributes healthy monounsaturated fats.

Caution:

- Watch portion sizes, as the mayonnaise and cheese can contribute to calorie intake.
- Adjust spice levels based on personal preference and sensitivity to heat.
- Choose whole-grain rice or quinoa for added nutritional benefits.

Mango Avocado Salsa Quinoa Bowl

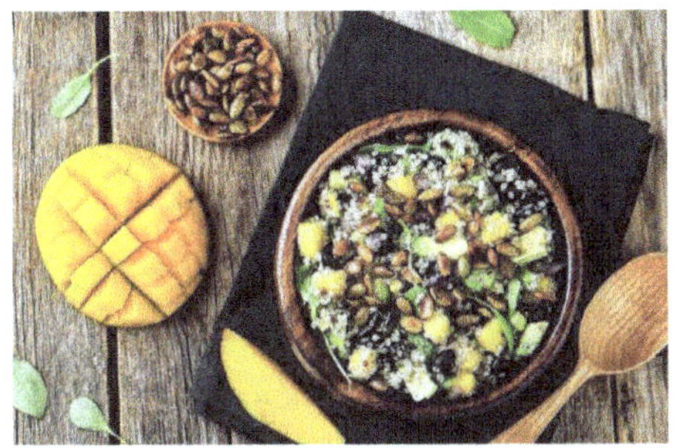

Ingredients:

- 1 cup quinoa, rinsed
- 2 cups water
- 1 ripe mango, diced
- 1 ripe avocado, diced
- 1/2 cup cherry tomatoes, halved
- 1/4 cup red onion, finely chopped
- 1/4 cup fresh cilantro, chopped
- Juice of 1 lime
- 2 tablespoons olive oil
- Salt and pepper to taste

Procedures:

- Cook Quinoa: In a medium saucepan, bring 2 cups of water to a boil. Add rinsed quinoa, reduce heat to low, cover, and simmer for 15-20 minutes or until quinoa is cooked and water is absorbed. Using a fork, fluff and set aside to cool.
- Prepare Salsa: In a large mixing bowl, combine diced mango, avocado, cherry tomatoes, red onion, and cilantro. Drizzle lime juice and olive oil over the mixture. Gently toss until well combined. Season with salt and pepper to taste.

- Assemble Bowl: In individual serving bowls, layer cooked quinoa as the base. Top with the mango avocado salsa mixture.
- Serve: Garnish with additional cilantro and lime wedges if desired. Serve immediately.

Time of Preparation:

- Approximately 30 minutes.

Tips and Tricks:

- Ensure the quinoa is properly rinsed to remove any bitterness.
- Dice the mango and avocado just before assembling to maintain freshness.
- Adjust lime juice and salt according to personal taste preferences.

Nutritional Value (per serving):

- Calories: Approximately 350-400 kcal
- Protein: 8g
- Fiber: 9g
- Healthy Fats: 15g
- Carbohydrates: 55g

Health Benefits:

- Quinoa provides a complete protein source.
- Mango and avocado offer vitamins, minerals, and healthy fats.
- High fiber content supports digestion.
- Rich in antioxidants from tomatoes, onion, and cilantro.

Caution:

- If allergic to any ingredients, substitute or omit accordingly.
- Moderation is key, especially for those watching calorie intake.

Sweet Potato and Blackberry Bowl

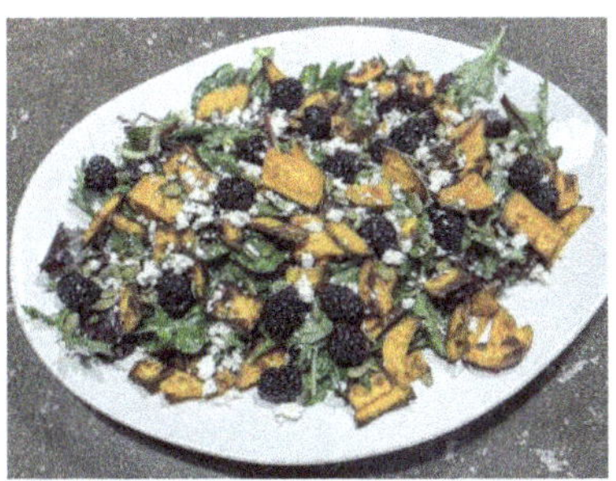

Ingredients:

- Diced and peeled two medium sweet potatoes
- 1 cup fresh blackberries
- 1/4 cup chopped pecans
- 2 tablespoons maple syrup
- 1 tablespoon coconut oil, melted
- 1 teaspoon cinnamon
- Pinch of salt

- For serving, Greek or coconut yogurt (optional).

Procedures:

- Roast Sweet Potatoes: Preheat the oven to 400°F (200°C). Toss diced sweet potatoes with melted coconut oil, maple syrup, cinnamon, and a pinch of salt Arrange them in a single layer on a baking sheet. Roast for 20-25 minutes or until sweet potatoes are tender and slightly caramelized.
- Prepare Blackberry Topping: In a small saucepan, warm the blackberries over medium heat for 3-4 minutes until they release their juices. Stir occasionally to prevent sticking. Remove from heat.
- Assemble Bowl: Divide the roasted sweet potatoes into serving bowls. Top with the warm blackberries, chopped pecans, and an additional drizzle of maple syrup if desired.

- Optional Yogurt: Serve the bowl with a dollop of Greek yogurt or coconut yogurt for added creaminess.

Time of Preparation:

- Approximately 30-35 minutes.

Tips and Tricks:

- Cut sweet potatoes into uniform sizes for even roasting.
- Adjust maple syrup and cinnamon according to your sweetness preference.
- Feel free to experiment with different nuts like walnuts or almonds.

Nutritional Value (per serving):

- Calories: Approximately 300-350 kcal
- Protein: 4g
- Healthy Fats: 12g
- Carbohydrates: 50g
- Fiber: 8g

Health Benefits:

- Sweet potatoes are high in antioxidants, fiber, and vitamins A and C.
- Blackberries provide vitamins, minerals, and antioxidants.
- Pecans contribute healthy fats, fiber, and essential nutrients.

Caution:

- Monitor portion sizes, especially for those watching calorie intake.
- Adjust ingredients to accommodate dietary restrictions or allergies.

Maple Cinnamon Apple Oat Bowl

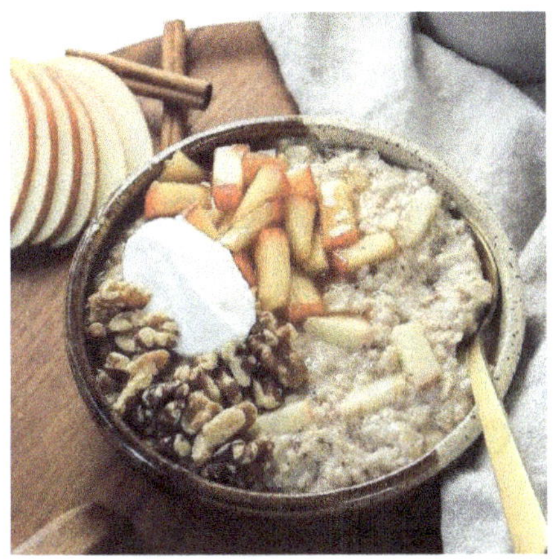

Ingredients:

- 1 cup rolled oats
- 1 3/4 cups almond milk (or any milk of your choice)
- 2 medium apples, peeled, cored, and diced
- 2 tablespoons pure maple syrup
- 1 teaspoon ground cinnamon
- 1/4 cup chopped walnuts or almonds (optional)

- For serving, Greek or coconut yogurt (optional).

Procedures:

- Prepare Oats: In a saucepan, combine rolled oats and almond milk. Bring over medium heat to a slow simmer. Stir occasionally and cook for 5-7 minutes or until oats are creamy and have absorbed the liquid.
- Sauté Apples: In a separate pan, sauté diced apples with a sprinkle of cinnamon over medium heat until they are softened but still have a slight crunch, about 4-5 minutes.
- Combine Oats and Apples: Add sautéed apples to the cooked oats. Mix in maple syrup and ground cinnamon. Stir well to combine.

- Optional Toppings: If desired, top the oatmeal with chopped nuts for added crunch. Serve with a dollop of Greek yogurt or coconut yogurt for extra creaminess.

Time of Preparation:

- Approximately 15-20 minutes.

Tips and Tricks:

- Use old-fashioned rolled oats for a hearty texture.

- Modify the sweetness by adjusting the maple syrup quantity.

- Try a variety of apple cultivars to get a range of flavors.

Nutritional Value (per serving):

- Calories: Approximately 350-400 kcal
- Protein: 8g
- Healthy Fats: 10g
- Carbohydrates: 65g
- Fiber: 10g

Health Benefits:

- Oats are a good source of fiber, aiding digestion and providing sustained energy.
- Apples contribute vitamins, minerals, and antioxidants.
- Cinnamon has anti-inflammatory properties and adds a warm flavor.

Caution:

- Be mindful of portion sizes, especially if watching calorie intake.
- Adjust ingredients to accommodate dietary preferences or restrictions.

7
Family-Friendly Bowls

Kid-Friendly Nut-Free Sunflower Seed Butter Bowl

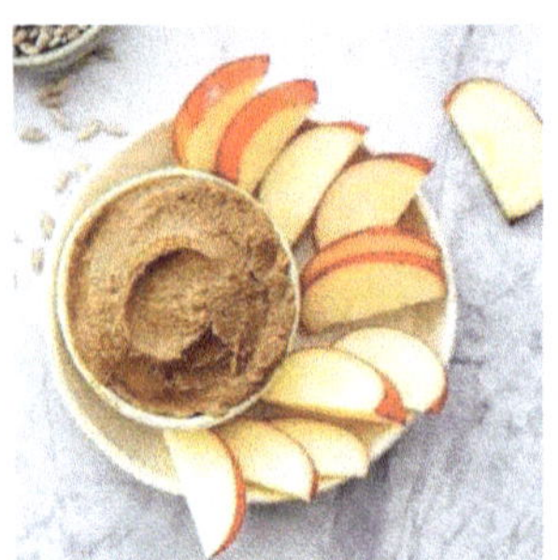

Ingredients:

- 1 cup sunflower seed butter
- 2 ripe bananas, sliced
- One cup of fresh raspberries, blueberries, or strawberries
- 1 tablespoon honey or maple syrup
- 1 teaspoon vanilla extract
- 1 cup granola
- 1 tablespoon chia seeds (optional)

Procedure:

- Prepare Sunflower Seed Butter: In a blender or food processor, blend sunflower seeds until they form a smooth butter-like consistency.
- Add honey or maple syrup and vanilla extract, blend until well combined.
- Assemble the Bowl: In a serving bowl, spread a generous layer of sunflower seed butter.
- Arrange sliced bananas and fresh berries on top.
- Top with Granola and Chia Seeds: Sprinkle granola evenly over the bowl for added crunch and nutrition.
- Optionally, sprinkle chia seeds for extra fiber and omega-3 fatty acids.
- Drizzle with Honey: Drizzle honey or maple syrup over the bowl for natural sweetness.

- Serve and Enjoy: Mix the ingredients together or let kids create their own combinations.

- Ensure the sunflower seed butter is at room temperature for easy spreading.
- Customize with kid-friendly toppings like mini chocolate chips or shredded coconut.
- Experiment with different berries for variety.

Nutritional Value per Serving:

- Calories: Approximately 400 calories
- Protein: 10g
- Fiber: 8g
- Healthy Fats: 20g
- Vitamin C: 15% DV
- Calcium: 6% DV
- Iron: 10% DV

Health Benefits:

- Sunflower seeds: High in magnesium, selenium, and vitamin E.
- Bananas: Rich in vitamin C and potassium.
- Berries: Rich in vitamin C and antioxidants.
- Granola: Provides fiber and energy-boosting carbohydrates.

Caution:

- Check the labels to ensure the sunflower seed butter is processed in a nut-free facility.
- Be aware of allergies; if anyone has a seed allergy, consult with a healthcare professional.
- Monitor portion sizes for calorie control.

Picky Eater Approved Hidden Veggie Bowl

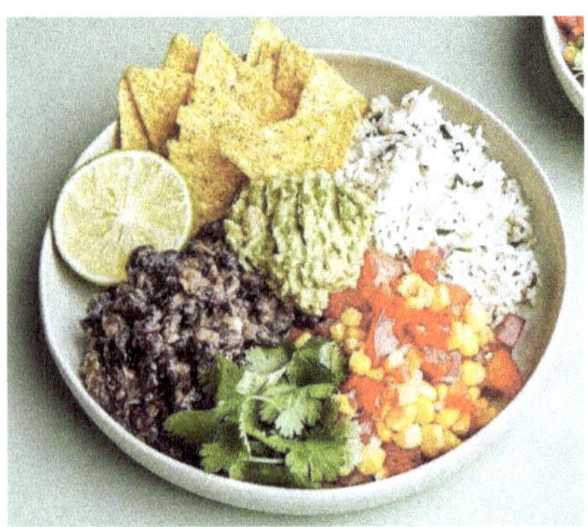

Ingredients:

- 1 cup quinoa or brown rice
- 1 cup finely grated carrots
- 1 cup finely chopped spinach
- 1 cup cherry tomatoes, halved
- 1 cup broccoli florets, steamed
- 1 cup cooked and shredded chicken or tofu
- 2 cloves garlic, minced
- 1 tablespoon olive oil
- 1 teaspoon dried herbs (oregano, basil, or thyme)
- Salt and pepper to taste
- Grated Parmesan cheese (optional)

Procedure:

- Cook Quinoa or Brown Rice: Prepare quinoa or brown rice according to package instructions.
- Saute Vegetables: In a pan, sauté minced garlic in olive oil until fragrant.
- Add grated carrots and chopped spinach, cook until softened.
- Incorporate halved cherry tomatoes and steamed broccoli florets.

- Add Protein: Mix in cooked and shredded chicken or tofu.
- Add salt, pepper, and dry herbs for seasoning.
- Combine with Quinoa or Brown Rice: Add the cooked quinoa or brown rice to the pan, mixing well to combine.
- Optional Topping: Sprinkle with grated Parmesan cheese for added flavor.
- Serve Warm: Dish out the Hidden Veggie Bowl while warm.

Tips and Tricks:

- Finely grate or chop veggies to make them less noticeable for picky eaters.
- Experiment with different veggies based on your child's preferences.
- Involve your child in the cooking process to increase their interest.

Nutritional Value per Serving:

- Calories: Approximately 350 calories
- Protein: 20g
- Fiber: 8g
- Vitamin A: 150% DV
- Vitamin C: 70% DV
- Iron: 15% DV
- Calcium: 10% DV

Health Benefits:

- Carrots: Rich in beta-carotene for eye health.
- Spinach: Rich in vital vitamins and iron.
- Broccoli: High in fiber and vitamin C.
- Quinoa or Brown Rice: Excellent sources of complex carbohydrates.

Caution:

- Be cautious of any allergies your child may have to specific vegetables.
- Monitor portion sizes based on your child's age and activity level.

- A thorough cooking of chicken is essential to prevent foodborne diseases.

Family Taco Night Fiesta Bowl

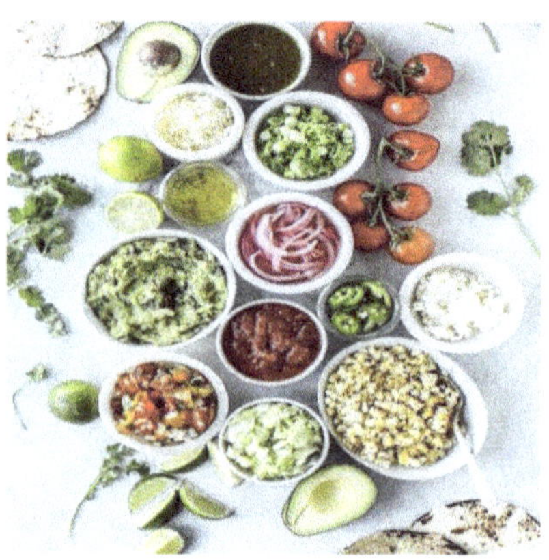

- 1 lb ground beef or ground turkey
- 1 packet taco seasoning
- One can of rinsed and drained black beans; one cup cooked brown rice or quinoa; and one cup fresh or frozen corn kernels
- 1 cup cherry tomatoes, diced
- 1 cup shredded lettuce
- 1 cup shredded cheddar cheese
- 1 avocado, sliced
- Salsa and sour cream for topping
- Fresh cilantro for garnish
- Tortilla chips for added crunch

- Cook Ground Meat: In a skillet, cook ground beef or turkey until browned.
- Drain excess fat and add taco seasoning according to packet instructions.

- Prepare Rice or Quinoa: Cook brown rice or quinoa as per package instructions.
- Assemble Bowl: In individual bowls, layer cooked rice or quinoa as the base.
- Add Toppings: Top with seasoned ground meat, black beans, corn, cherry tomatoes, lettuce, and shredded cheese.
- Garnish and Serve: Garnish with avocado slices, salsa, sour cream, and fresh cilantro.
- Serve with tortilla chips on the side for added texture.

Tips and Tricks:

- Customize toppings based on family preferences.
- Set up a taco bar for a fun and interactive family dinner.
- Warm tortilla shells for those who prefer traditional tacos.

Nutritional Value per Serving:

- Calories: Approximately 500 calories
- Protein: 25g
- Fiber: 10g
- Vitamin C: 20% DV
- Calcium: 20% DV
- Iron: 25% DV

Health Benefits:

- Lean Protein: Ground beef or turkey provides essential proteins.
- Whole Grains: Brown rice or quinoa for fiber and complex carbohydrates.
- Vegetables: A variety of veggies contribute essential vitamins and minerals.
- Healthy Fats: Avocado adds monounsaturated fats.

Caution:

- Be mindful of any dietary restrictions or allergies within the family.
- Control sodium content by choosing a low-sodium taco seasoning or making your own.
- Monitor portion sizes to maintain a balanced meal.

8

Dessert Bowls

Chocolate Banana Smoothie Bowl

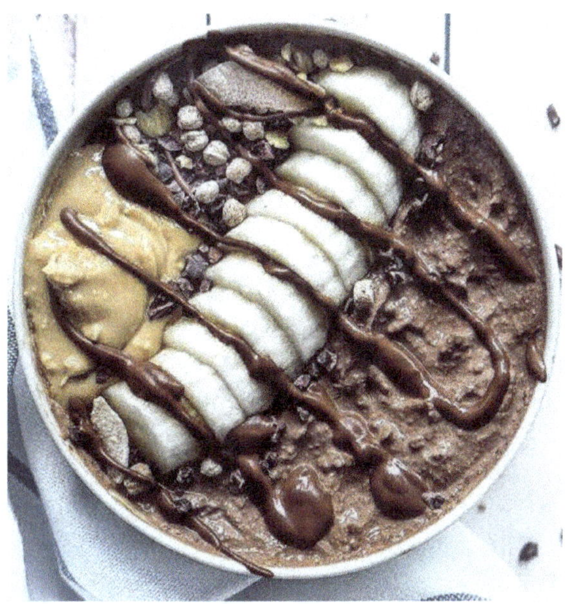

- 2 ripe bananas, frozen
- 1/2 cup Greek yogurt
- 1/4 cup almond milk (or any milk of your choice)
- 2 tablespoons unsweetened cocoa powder
- 1 tablespoon honey or maple syrup
- 1/4 teaspoon vanilla extract
- Toppings: sliced bananas, strawberries, chia seeds, granola, dark chocolate shavings

Procedure:

- Peel and slice the ripe bananas before freezing them for a few hours or overnight.
- In a blender, combine the frozen banana slices, Greek yogurt, almond milk, cocoa powder, honey or maple syrup, and vanilla extract.
- Blend until creamy and smooth, adding extra milk as necessary to modify the consistency.

- Approximately 10 minutes, excluding freezing time for bananas.

Tips and Tricks:

- Add frozen berries for an extra burst of flavor and a thicker consistency.
- Customize toppings based on personal preferences for added texture and nutritional benefits.

Nutritional Value per Serving:

- (Note: Values are approximate and may vary based on specific ingredients and quantities used)
- Calories: 300
- Protein: 12g
- Fat: 5g
- Carbohydrates: 55g
- Fiber: 8g
- Sugar: 30g

Health Benefits:

- Rich in Antioxidants: Cocoa powder is loaded with antioxidants, contributing to overall health.
- Protein Boost: Greek yogurt provides a protein boost, aiding in muscle repair and maintenance.
- Good Fats: Almond milk adds healthy fats, promoting heart health.

Caution:

- Monitor portion sizes, especially if watching calorie intake.
- Be mindful of added sweeteners; adjust according to personal preferences and dietary needs.

- Individuals with allergies should substitute ingredients accordingly.

Berry Bliss Acai Bowl

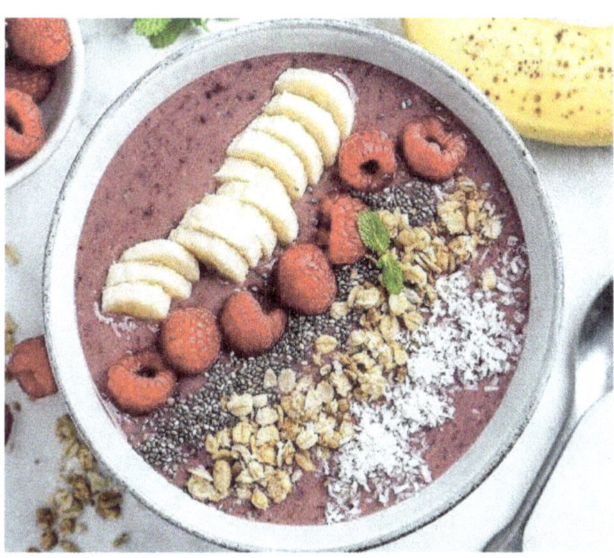

- 1 packet frozen Acai puree (unsweetened)
- 1 frozen banana
- 1/2 cup almond milk (or any other type of milk of your choice) • 1/2 cup mixed berries (strawberries, blueberries, and raspberries)
- One tablespoon agave syrup or honey
- Granola, coconut flakes, cut strawberries, chia seeds, and honey drizzled over top

- Soften the frozen Acai packet by running it under warm water for a short while.
- In a blender, combine the Acai puree, frozen banana, mixed berries, almond milk, and honey or agave syrup.
- Blend until smooth and creamy, adjusting the thickness with more milk if needed.

- Approximately 10 minutes, excluding Acai packet thawing time.

- Add a handful of spinach or kale for a nutritional boost without altering the taste.
- If you want your consistency to be thicker, use frozen fruits.
- Experiment with different toppings to add texture and flavor variety.

Nutritional Value per Serving:

- (Values are an estimate that might change depending on the precise components and amounts utilized.)
- Calories: 250
- Protein: 5g
- Fat: 10g
- Carbohydrates: 40g
- Fiber: 8g
- Sugar: 20g

Health Benefits:

- Antioxidant-Rich Acai: Acai berries are packed with antioxidants, supporting immune health.
- Fiber Boost: Berries and toppings contribute to a high-fiber content, aiding digestion.
- Omega-3 Fatty Acids: Chia seeds provide essential omega-3s, promoting heart health.

Caution:

- Be mindful of portion sizes, especially if incorporating sweetened toppings.
- Check the Acai packet for added sugars and opt for unsweetened versions for a healthier bowl.
- Those with nut allergies can choose a milk alternative without compromising flavor.

Coconut Mango Rice Pudding Bowl

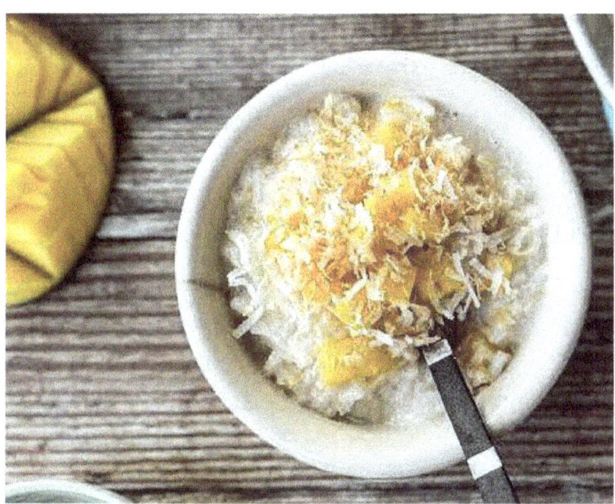

- 1 cup jasmine rice
- 2 cups coconut milk
- 1/4 cup sugar (adjust to taste)
- 1/2 teaspoon vanilla extract
- 1 ripe mango, diced
- 1/4 cup shredded coconut, toasted
- Optional toppings: sliced almonds, mint leaves

Procedure:

- Use cold water to rinse the jasmine rice until the water turns clear.
- In a saucepan, combine the rinsed rice, coconut milk, sugar, and vanilla extract.
- Bring the mixture to a simmer over medium heat, then reduce to low and cover. Cook for 20-25 minutes, or until the rice is tender and has absorbed most of the liquid.
- Allow the rice pudding to cool slightly. Stir in the diced mango.
- Divide the pudding into bowls and top with toasted shredded coconut, sliced almonds, and mint leaves.

- Approximately 30 minutes, excluding cooling time.

Tips and Tricks:

- Use light coconut milk for a lighter version or full-fat for a richer flavor.
- Experiment with different rice varieties for varied textures.
- Adjust sugar to your liking; ripe mangoes add natural sweetness.

Nutritional Value per Serving:

- (Values are an estimate that might change depending on the precise components and amounts utilized.)
- Calories: 300
- Protein: 3g
- Fat: 10g
- Carbohydrates: 50g
- Fiber: 2g
- Sugar: 20g

Health Benefits:

- Rich in Healthy Fats: Coconut milk provides medium-chain triglycerides (MCTs), known for various health benefits.
- Vitamins and Minerals: Mangoes are a great source of vitamins A and C, contributing to skin health and immune function.
- Energy Boost: The combination of rice and coconut offers sustained energy.

Caution:

- Monitor sugar intake, especially if aiming for a lower-sugar diet.
- Consider portion sizes, as rice pudding can be calorie-dense.
- Individuals with rice allergies should choose an alternative grain.

Embracing a Plant-Based Lifestyle

Embracing a plant-based lifestyle involves adopting a diet and way of living that primarily revolves around plant-derived foods while minimizing or eliminating animal products. This choice extends beyond just food, encompassing various aspects of daily life. Here's a detailed exploration of the key elements of embracing a plant-based lifestyle:

Nutrient-Rich Diet:

- Whole Plant Foods: Focus on consuming a variety of fruits, vegetables, whole grains, nuts, and legumes. These foods provide essential nutrients, fiber, and antioxidants crucial for overall well-being.
- Protein Sources: Incorporate plant-based protein sources such as beans, lentils, tofu, tempeh, and plant-based protein powders to ensure adequate protein intake.
- Healthy Fats: Opt for sources like avocados, nuts, seeds, and olive oil for healthy fats that support cardiovascular health.
- Vitamins and Minerals: Pay attention to obtaining sufficient vitamins B12, D, iron, calcium, and omega-3 fatty acids, which can be sourced from fortified foods or supplements.

Environmental Impact:

- Reduced Carbon Footprint: Plant-based diets generally have a lower environmental impact as they require fewer natural resources and produce fewer greenhouse gas emissions compared to animal agriculture.
- Sustainable Practices: Embrace locally sourced and seasonal produce to further reduce the environmental impact of your food choices.

Ethical Considerations:

- Animal Welfare: Choosing plant-based options aligns with the ethical stance of avoiding harm to animals. This lifestyle promotes compassion towards animals and supports cruelty-free practices.

Health Benefits:

- Heart Health: Plant-based diets are associated with lower risks of heart disease, high blood pressure, and cholesterol levels, contributing to better cardiovascular health.
- Weight Management: Many plant-based foods are naturally lower in calories and saturated fats, making it easier to maintain a healthy weight.
- Disease Prevention: Studies suggest that a plant-based lifestyle may reduce the risk of certain diseases, including type 2 diabetes and certain types of cancers.

- Diverse Cuisine: Embracing a plant-based lifestyle opens the door to a rich tapestry of global cuisines, encouraging creativity in the kitchen with inventive and delicious plant-based recipes.
- Plant-Based Alternatives: Explore the growing market of plant-based alternatives for traditional animal products, such as plant-based burgers, dairy-free milk, and vegan cheeses.

Social and Community Aspects:

- Community Engagement: Connect with like-minded individuals through local or online plant-based communities. Share experiences, recipes, and tips for a supportive network.
- Educational Outreach: Share your knowledge and experiences with others to promote awareness about the benefits of a plant-based lifestyle, contributing to a positive impact on the community.

Mindful Eating:

- Conscious Choices: Embrace mindfulness in your food choices, considering the impact on your health, the environment, and ethical considerations.
- Balanced Nutrition: Ensure a well-balanced and varied diet to meet your nutritional needs, paying attention to a mix of different plant foods.

Embracing a plant-based lifestyle is a holistic approach that intertwines personal health, environmental sustainability, and ethical considerations. It's a journey towards a more compassionate, mindful, and sustainable way of living.

Plant-Based Power Bowls

Plant-based power bowls are vibrant, nutrient-packed meals that showcase a variety of plant foods in a visually appealing and delicious way. These bowls are not only a feast for the eyes but also a powerhouse of essential nutrients. Let's delve into the key components and benefits of plant-based power bowls:

Base:

- Whole Grains: Start with a base of nutrient-dense whole grains like quinoa, brown rice, farro, or bulgur. These grains provide complex carbohydrates and fiber for sustained energy.

- Legumes: Include a variety of legumes such as chickpeas, black beans, lentils, or edamame for a plant-based protein boost.
- Tofu or Tempeh: Grilled or sautéed tofu or tempeh adds a satisfying texture and protein richness to the bowl.

Colorful Vegetables:

- Dark Leafy Greens: Incorporate nutrient-rich greens like kale, spinach, or Swiss chard for a dose of vitamins, minerals, and antioxidants.
- Colorful Veggies: Include a rainbow of vegetables such as bell peppers, cherry tomatoes, cucumbers, carrots, and beets to enhance both flavor and nutritional diversity.

Healthy Fats:

- Avocado: Sliced avocado contributes creamy texture and heart-healthy monounsaturated fats.
- Nuts and Seeds: Sprinkle a handful of seeds (sunflower, pumpkin, sesame) or nuts (almonds, walnuts) for added crunch and omega-3 fatty acids.
- Drizzle of Olive Oil: A light drizzle of extra-virgin olive oil not only enhances flavor but also provides essential fats.

Flavorful Dressings and Sauces:

- Tahini Dressing: A blend of tahini, lemon juice, garlic, and water creates a creamy and tangy dressing.
- Balsamic Glaze or Soy-Ginger Sauce: Add depth to the bowl with a drizzle of balsamic glaze or a flavorful soy-ginger sauce.

Extras for Texture:

- Crispy Toppings: Add crunch with toppings like roasted chickpeas, crispy shallots, or baked tortilla strips.
- Fresh Herbs: Garnish with fresh herbs such as cilantro, parsley, or mint for a burst of flavor.

- Personalized Touch: Customize your power bowl based on personal preferences and dietary needs. Experiment with different ingredients to keep things exciting.
- Health Benefits:
- Nutrient Density: Plant-based power bowls are packed with vitamins, minerals, and antioxidants, supporting overall health and well-being.
- Dietary Fiber: The combination of whole grains, vegetables, and legumes ensures an ample supply of dietary fiber, promoting digestive health and satiety.
- Balanced Nutrition: These bowls provide a well-rounded mix of macronutrients, including carbohydrates, proteins, and healthy fats, contributing to sustained energy levels.

Culinary Creativity:

- Global Inspirations: Draw inspiration from various cuisines worldwide to create diverse and flavorful plant-based power bowls.
- Seasonal Variations: Embrace seasonal produce to keep your bowls fresh, exciting, and in harmony with nature's offerings.

Plant-based power bowls are not just a meal; they are a celebration of flavors, textures, and nutrients. Whether you're a seasoned chef or a novice in the kitchen, crafting your own plant-based power bowl allows for endless creativity and a delightful culinary experience.

CONCLUSION

In the annals of culinary evolution, the emergence of Plant-Based Power Bowls stands as a glorious chapter, heralding a transformative era where gastronomy intertwines with health, sustainability, and sheer culinary ingenuity. These vibrant bowls, akin to a Renaissance masterpiece, paint a canvas of colors, flavors, and nourishment, rewriting the narrative of what a truly satisfying and wholesome meal entails.

As we reflect upon the historical tapestry of our dietary choices, the Plant-Based Power Bowl emerges as a culinary luminary, illuminating the path towards a healthier, more compassionate future. This gastronomic revolution echoes the wisdom of ages, harkening back to a time when civilizations revered the bounty of the earth and celebrated the artistry of combining diverse ingredients.

Much like an ancient mosaic, these bowls intricately piece together elements from various corners of the plant kingdom — the resilient grains, the verdant greens, the protein-rich legumes, and the luxurious embrace of healthy fats. Each bowl, a testament to the culmination of culinary knowledge, reflects a harmonious synergy between taste and nutrition.

In the grand theater of dietary choices, the Plant-Based Power Bowl takes center stage, not merely as a fleeting trend but as a timeless masterpiece. Its legacy is etched in the annals of progressive dining, challenging norms, and inviting all to partake in the symphony of flavors orchestrated by nature itself.

As we savor the present, let us recognize the historical significance of the Plant-Based Power Bowl — a culinary renaissance that honors the planet, respects our fellow beings, and elevates the act of nourishing oneself to an art form. In its wholesome embrace, we find a convergence of gastronomic delight, healthful living, and a profound connection to the earth's abundance.

And so, with each forkful, we not only nourish our bodies but also contribute to a narrative where the pursuit of wellness aligns with culinary excellence. The Plant-Based Power Bowl, an immortal chapter in our gastronomic history, beckons us to savor the flavors of a more enlightened era, where the plate becomes a canvas, and every meal is a masterpiece.